LIVE
FAST
LOSE
WEIGHT

LIVE
FAST
LOSE
WEIGHT

CHARLOTTE
CROSBY

headline

First published in 2016 by HEADLINE PUBLISHING GROUP

1

Cataloguing in Publication Data is available from the British Library.

ISBN 978 1 4722 3198 7

Recipes created by Louisa Carter and Charlotte Simpkins
Additional recipe advice by David Souter
Project edited by Emma Tait
Design and art direction by Lynne Eve, Design Jam
Photography by Haarala Hamilton
Food styling by Kat Mead
Hair and make-up by Cassie Lomas
Styling by Lorraine McCullough
Props styling by Jemima Hetherington
Dietetic Input by Azmina Govindji RD
Management by Kate O'Shea, Bold Management

All photographs © Haarala Hamilton except page 6 © Ewelina Stechnij, page 19 © Yeamake/Shutterstock;
page 26 © Ewelina Stechnij; page 32 © Nazzu/Shutterstock; page 33 © mutation/Shutterstock;
page 58 © Ewelina Stechnij; page 64 © Ewelina Stechnij and page 80 © Ewelina Stechnij.

Printed and bound in Germany by Mohn Media

HEADLINE PUBLISHING GROUP
An Hachette UK Company
Carmelite House
50 Victoria Embankment
London EC4 0DZ

www.headline.co.uk
www.hachette.co.uk

Neither this diet nor any other diet programme should be followed without first consulting a
healthcare professional. If you have any special conditions requiring attention, you should consult
with your healthcare professional regularly regarding possible modification of the programme
contained in this book.

CONTENTS

MY STORY

Oh, hiya! I bet you never thought this would happen. No, not just me writing a book – I've done that, which surprised me as much as anyone (well, maybe my old English teacher was a bit more surprised). But me writing a book about… wait for it, drum roll please … living a healthy lifestyle.

I know. I almost can't believe it either!

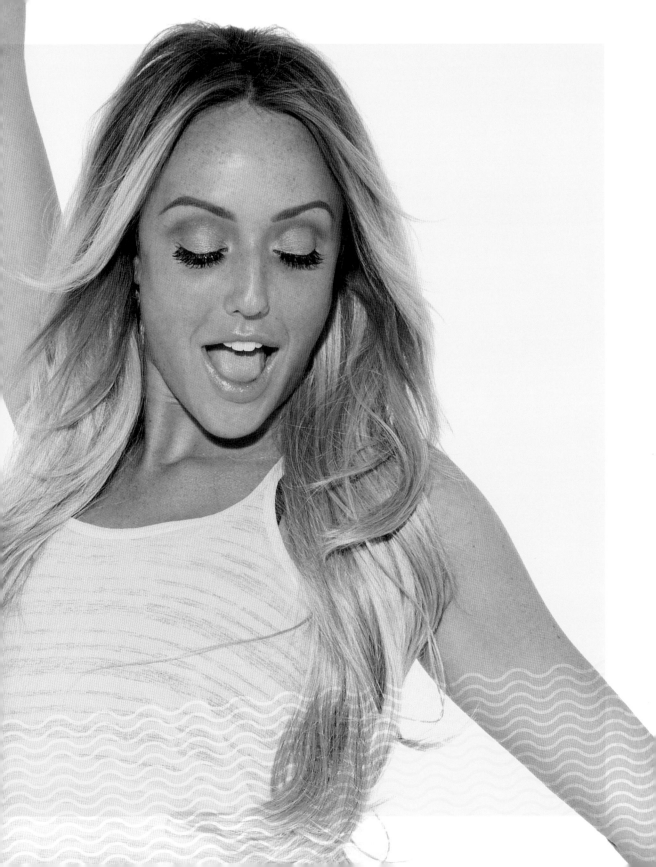

Let's look at the facts. I'm Charlotte Letitia Crosby, I'm 25 and I'm the girl who was almost rejected from *Geordie Shore* because the MTV producers thought my drunken stories were too outrageous to be true. Well, if you read my autobiography *Me Me Me* you'll know just how wrong they were. So, all things considered, you might not have had me down as one of the boring lettuce-and-sipping-on-a-soft-drink-at-a-party types.

And you'd be right. I'm not.

What I *am* is someone who's managed to totally transform my body and – more importantly – how I feel. And I've done it all while still going out and partying (and getting mortal – but that's never a good idea so you shouldn't copy that bit!). Why should you care? Because you can too.

I want to get you feeling good, looking great – and having an amazing time in the process. Not, when all your friends are going out for a meal and drinks, having to say, 'Oh, I can't come, girls. I'm trying to lose weight.' I certainly don't do that – I'm in *Geordie Shore*! I go in that house and I have a great time for six weeks. I do carry on working out when I'm in there, but not as hard and I eat sensibly (when I'm sober!). So, yes, when I come out I don't feel as fit, but I haven't put all the weight back on. That's also because I do the work before I go in there, and I do the work when I come out. And that doesn't mean that when I'm out of the house I'm secretly living like a nun. Let's face it I'm 25 and I'm single so of course I go out and party – but I've got some great hangover tips (I'll tell you about those later).

A lot of people think that losing weight and being healthy is about being strict and having no life. I've proved it's not about that – it's about having a balance. In fact, I'm feeling so inspired about all this that I might even write a little poem, just to celebrate this moment we're sharing…

Welcome to my recipe book!

If you wanna lose weight, have a little look.

Have fun, go wild and still have cheats.

I know what you're thinking, this sounds a treat!

Have you ever thought diets are dull,

I wanna have fun, live life to the full?

Well, stop the wishing, there's no need to pray,

It's time to get fit and lose weight the Charlotte way!

Hope you enjoyed that. Anyway, talking about balance – I'd lost mine.

You've probably already seen that photo of me on the beach in a bikini back in June 2014. Now obviously I didn't love that bikini photo. But when I look at it now, I know it served a purpose. Because everyone needs something that makes them think, 'Wow. I'm going to do something about this.' And that photo's what kick-started me to lose more than two-and-a-half stone in nine months.

At my heaviest, I was eleven stone five. With my height and build, I just looked *swollen* everywhere. I didn't even think about what size I was buying, I'd just buy large, baggy things. At the end of those nine months, by March 2015, I was down to eight stone nine and a size six. Along the way I made my fitness DVD *Charlotte Crosby's 3 Minute Belly Blitz*, which covered a really important aspect of how I did it – exercise – but not the rest of it.

In this book, I'm going to tell you about all the other aspects of my healthy lifestyle: how to have a great night out without wrecking your hard work, my go-to snacks and swaps, my favourite cheat meals (and why it's *okay* to cheat!), all my motivational tricks to get you fired up about what's ahead and my number-one tip for making this way of living work for you. Most important of all, I'm going to give you all my go-to healthy recipes that I make day in, day out, when I'm at home. That's my favourite breakfasts, my filling (but not fattening) lunches and dinners, and my tasty smoothies and shakes. I've even got lovely cocktails and puddings that won't ruin your hard work! Don't ever say I'm not nice to you…

But first, I'd better explain how I ended up turning my lifestyle around to start with.

BODY TALK

Growing up, I never really had a problem with my body image. For girls in school today, it seems like it's all about looking good. But I never really thought about it, it never crossed my mind. I loved my food, so me mam never had to force us to eat, or force us to eat vegetables – I just ate whatever, whenever, proper home cooking. We always had sweets in the house but I just didn't really like them. When I found the weight creeping on, when I was a lot older – about 23, 24 – that was the first time I'd felt not quite right in myself.

Looking back, I can see why I was getting bigger. On *Geordie Shore*, everyone loved me for who I was, and I didn't have to be anyone else – which was great! – but what that also meant was that I got *really* comfortable. And life in the house meant there was plenty of opportunity for me to eat unhealthy foods and go mad with the booze. I'd be spending weeks at a time in there, getting mortal every night, then eating hangover food the next day. When I wasn't in the house, there'd be PAs – personal appearances – and events where I could carry on in the same way.

I did try to lose weight once – I lost seven pounds through exercise and cutting out crap from my diet – but then I got with my ex, Mitch, and I just didn't bother anymore. When you've got a boyfriend you get so relaxed, don't you? He didn't really mind what I looked like, anyway. If I did notice that I was getting bigger, I'd just put it to the back of my mind and try not to think about it. The truth was, of course, I *did* think about it because I'd want to wear nice things on a night out and I felt like I just looked fat in everything. It did get me down. But as much as I could, I tried to put it out of my head.

MAM KNOWS BEST

At least I did until that photo woke me up. That and Letitia Crosby. Letitia's me mam. She's a brilliant mam, I love her so much. When she started to get on my back about my weight a lot, that was the other turning point. It got to the stage where I'd get off a flight after a PA, where I'd have been drinking pints of creamy Baileys (that *might* have something to do with why I was gaining so much weight!), I'd have some fast food in the airport, then I'd get in the car. There she'd be – me mam – sitting there, looking at my belly. 'Oh,' she'd say. 'Getting bigger, isn't it?' In that raised-eyebrow way.

And I hated her for it! I'd think, 'You're such a bad mam! You are an awful mam to be saying such horrible things about your daughter and making us feel so low.' I would go to my friends and cry about it. From anyone else? I would not give a shit. I've got nearly three million followers on Twitter and I'd get comments off them about me being 'fat' – and much worse than that – all the time. I do not care about something written on a computer screen from someone I don't even know. But when it was coming from me mam? It would get me down. She'd always try to get me to eat healthily when I was home.

'You want a piece of chicken for dinner? You want a piece of salmon?'

'Er, no,' I'd say. I didn't want that, I just wanted junk food all the time.

But now, when I think back to it, her letting me know that I needed to change my lifestyle was the best thing that she could have done, because it was her who made me think, 'I'm doing this now, I'm doing it for myself – and to prove to you I can!' I know she only had my best interests at heart – she just wanted me to look after myself. It's funny to think how much I've changed since then.

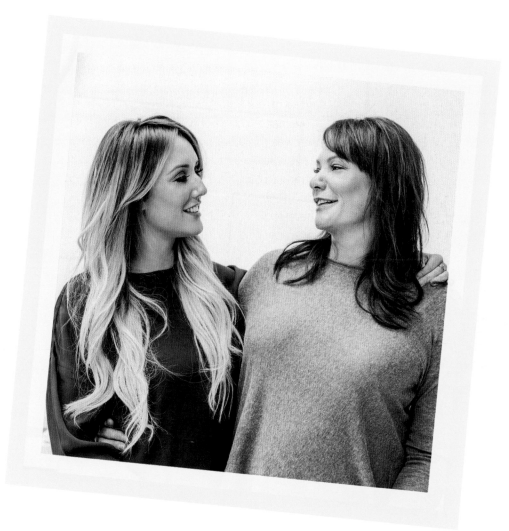

Now, I'll cook all my healthy recipes for me mam and dad, and they love it. They've jumped on the bandwagon! Me mam's even doing my exercise DVD herself and she's lost a bit of weight already. Go on Mam!

IT'S...
SUPER CHARLOTTE

Maybe you're still thinking, 'Ah, that sounds great, but why should I bother?' Let me tell you. As much as I like being able to wear whatever I want these days, it's not even about how I look – I'm happy about how I *feel*. After changing me diet and starting to exercise, the plusses, for me, are all about being fitter and being able to do more.

I'll give you an example. When I'm in *Geordie Shore*, just down the road from the house we live in there's a room where we film green-screen scenes (where we talk to the camera about what's going on). We get pulled out of the house to do them all the time. Now, when I was bigger, I would never run down there because I'd get so out of breath. 'I'm not going to bother, I'm going to walk it,' I'd tell myself. But now? These days, I'm sprinting down to green screen, I'm sprinting back and I'm not even puffing! Funny as it sounds, I'm so proud of myself. And life is full of nice little moments like that.

I feel different in myself, too. When I was a lot bigger, I always felt lethargic, tired, I didn't want to do things – everything was a hassle and a chore. When you're healthy, it's the opposite of that: you've got so much energy, you feel up for anything. So eating well makes you feel just great mentally too.

★

CHARLOTTE'S
WORDS OF WISDOM

EMOTIONAL EATING

I used to do this – eating because of how I felt, not because I was hungry – all the time when I was bigger. If I got down, the first thing I'd do was go round to my mate's and we'd order a Chinese. And if you are upset and food's what makes you feel better? So be it. But now I don't comfort eat because I've changed. And you will too. Once you're into this lifestyle, and you see results, it becomes part of your life and you won't turn to food when you're fed up.

Yes, it can be tough. I've had my low moments. I've wanted to eat my favourite unhealthy foods – and not just save them for a cheat meal – and join in when all my friends were getting kebabs and chips on nights out. Sometimes I've found the exercise pretty hard, too. I'd think, 'Why am I doing this to myself?' But when I think back on it all, I feel amazing, really proud of what I've achieved – all the low points were worth it.

And don't forget the high points. I'll happily admit I loved all the compliments I got when I got healthy. Even Cheryl Cole (as she was then) complimented me! I bumped into her when I was doing some filming for *The Xtra Factor*. She was having her photo taken and looked absolutely beautiful, I was in awe. Then she spotted me:

'Oh hiya, Charlotte!'

'Fuck me,' I thought. 'Cheryl Cole's talking to us.'

'Hiya Cheryl, how are you?' I said, all breezy.

'How are you? You're looking great!' she replied.

'Wow,' I thought. 'Cheryl Cole just gave us a compliment!
This is amazing, the best day ever.'

And Gary from *Geordie Shore*, who I've been on and off with over the years, told me: 'Charlotte, you look like series one Charlotte,' which was when I was dead skinny. And he started fancying us again… but I cared more about Cheryl!

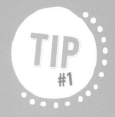

CHARLOTTE'S LIVE FAST LOSE WEIGHT ★TIP★

And speaking of Cheryl, there's nothing like listening to some motivating music when you're exercising. Her *Fight For This Love* is great for getting you going in the gym. This is what I like listening to, to inspire me:

☆ Martin Garrix / *Animals*

This is a good one for building momentum.

☆ Livvi Franc / *Now I'm That Bitch*

We used to listen to this one when we were getting ready, but I do think it makes you feel like you are the shit, so you get dead cocky in your workout and push yourself harder!

☆ Becky G / *Break a Sweat*

For obvious reasons.

☆ Katy Perry / *California Gurls*

Because she talks about being skinny and wearing hot pants and I like to imagine that's what I'll be doing on a beach on holiday, so this song helps me to work towards that.

☆ Justin Bieber / *What Do You Mean?*

This is just an absolute tune – working out or not, it has to be in there.

☆ Fergie / *Fergalicious*

I love the lines about being fit and going to the gym.

☆ Pussycat Dolls / *Buttons*

This is a really sexy song.

☆ Beyoncé / *Upgrade You*

Any Beyoncé song is a girl-power-be-strong song! So this is great one to feel empowered to.

GETTING STARTED

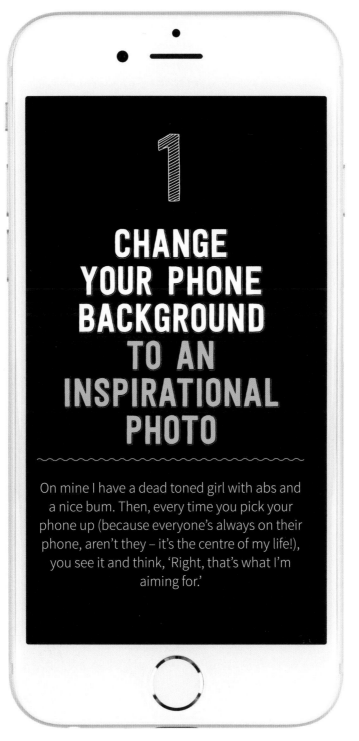

1

CHANGE YOUR PHONE BACKGROUND TO AN INSPIRATIONAL PHOTO

On mine I have a dead toned girl with abs and a nice bum. Then, every time you pick your phone up (because everyone's always on their phone, aren't they – it's the centre of my life!), you see it and think, 'Right, that's what I'm aiming for.'

GO ON A HEALTHY FOOD SHOP.
MAKE IT YOUR MISSION!

Start by making a list – write down all the healthy foods you want to get. Then go to the supermarket and buy your broccoli, your stir-fry vegetables, carrots and hummus, all your protein – your chicken, your mince – and pack your fridge full. It's exciting to think, 'I'm going to start afresh.' You can see my store-cupboard shopping list on page 82.

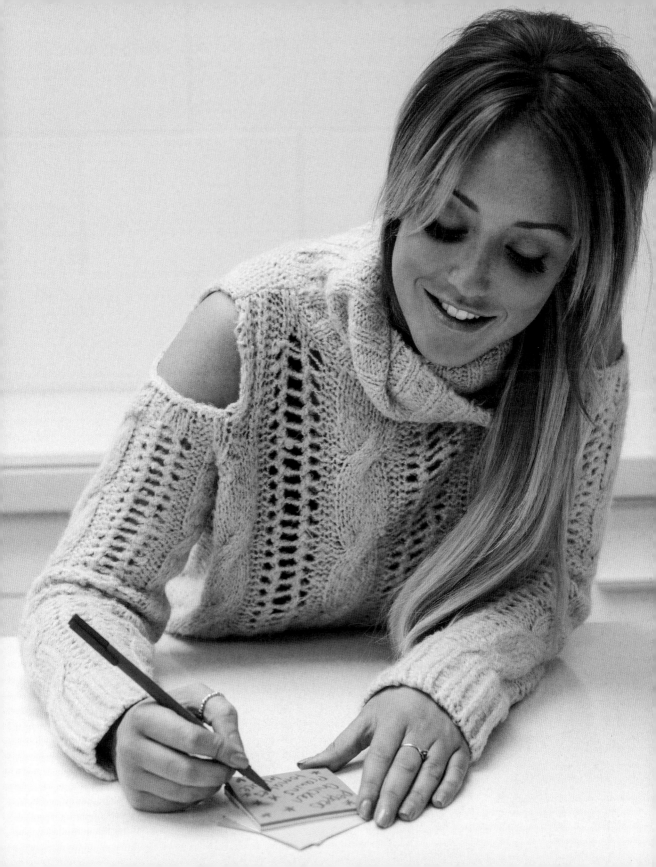

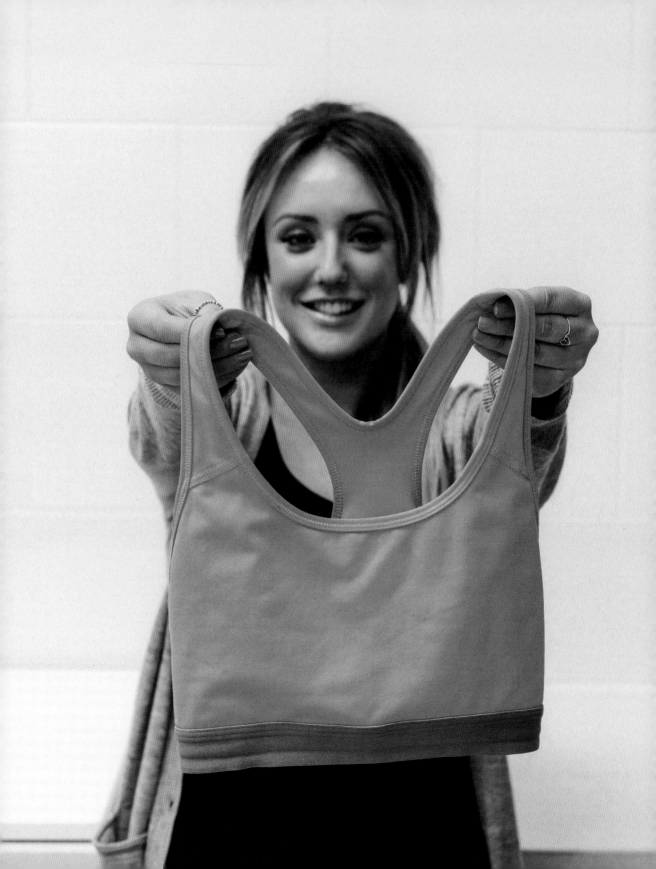

GO OUT AND GET YOURSELF SOME REALLY NICE WORKOUT GEAR

Loads of bright, nice stuff, so you're excited to wear it to the gym. It gets you motivated. (I'll tell you exactly what I like in a bit.)

STAY IN THE SHOPS –
THERE'S SOMETHING ELSE
YOU'VE GOT TO BUY

Find a dress that you love… and buy it in the size you want to be. Now I know what you're saying: 'No, never, not in a small', or whatever size you're aiming for. But I've done this myself. I went to Zara and I bought a dress in size small – a lovely little peach thing – and even on the hanger it was too tiny: when I held it up against me it didn't even cover me. I hung it in my wardrobe, and I'd look at that dress and think, 'NO WAY. No way am I ever going to get in that.' It seemed such a wild dream – so far away from my reality – it was almost unachievable.

Nine months later, when I'd lost the weight, I remembered it. 'Shit! I forgot about the dress.' I went to my wardrobe, tried it on… and it was too big. I needed an extra small! I was buzzing. So go out there and buy that dress and tell yourself: 'I will fit in that dress. I am going to wear that dress, and I will look GREAT.'

TAKE PHOTOS OF YOURSELF AS YOU ARE AT THE BEGINNING

From the front, from the side and from the back – you can just use your phone and a full-length mirror. And then make sure you keep taking them – once a month is more than enough – once you've got going. You can actually see your body changing. It's great motivation, because you can track your progress so clearly. When I was losing weight, I took pictures a lot and used an app so I could line them up in a gallery, next to each other. Every two months – so I'd wait a decent amount of time – I'd take a new set of photos to add. Seeing the difference between each new set of photos and the last made me so excited about what I could achieve by the time I took the next lot.

MY LIFE-STYLE

There's one thing people always want to ask me (and no, it's not how big Gary from *Geordie Shore*'s 'parsnip' is). It's, 'What's your diet, what do you eat?' And to that I'd just say, 'You already know what to eat!'

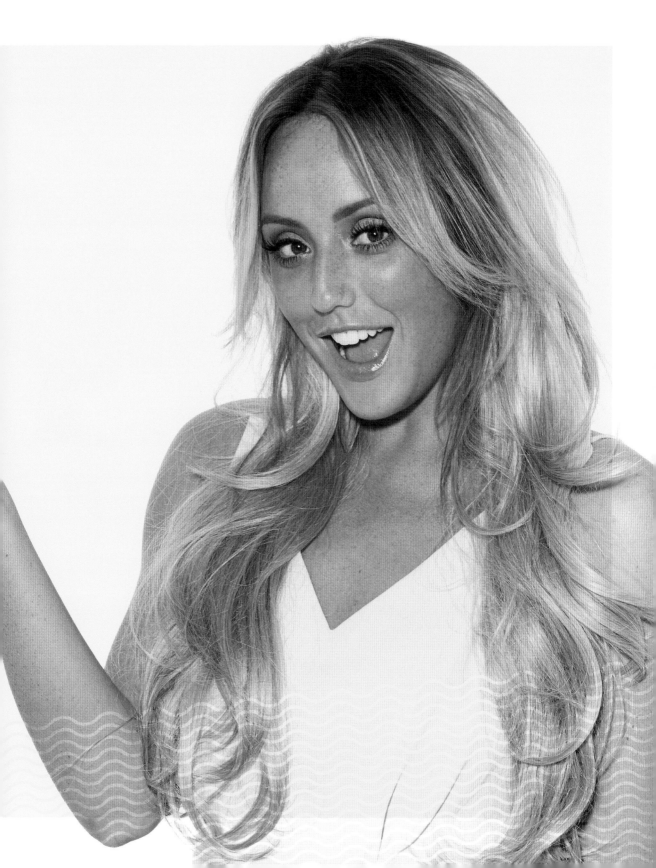

I knew what to eat, even when I was at my biggest. Everyone knows. It's simple: it's protein – meat, fish, eggs and beans – and it's vegetables. It's not a lot of crisps and cake and rubbish. And you're taught that from a young age. So when people ask me, I say: 'I eat healthily. What do you think is healthy?'

'Well…' they reply, 'chicken and vegetables.'

'Right,' I say. 'That's what I eat!' It's not rocket science. People think that there's some kind of magic secret, but there's no magic secret, there's no fad diet that's going to work for you long term – it's about being healthy.

Why protein – and, er, what exactly is it? You find lots of protein in meat, chicken, fish, eggs, dairy products like milk and yoghurt, beans, lentils and nuts. It fills you up and helps repair and build your muscles – as well as being used by your body in a ton of other ways. As for the veg, we all know that eating your veggies gives you the vitamins and minerals that help you feel and look good. They also give you a bit of protein and carbs.

Carbs – carbohydrates, if we're being proper about it – are another essential, giving your body energy. There are both starches and sugars (here's a clue – anything sweet's probably got more of the last one). Starchy high-carb foods include bread, pasta, rice, potatoes, oats and grains – but they're easy to overeat! And if you're not using that energy, your body's eventually going to store it as fat. As for sugary foods, they're trickier – they give you a big burst of energy all at once, then your body is left craving more… and you can get into that trap of repeat trips to the biscuit tin.

I normally only eat high-carb foods on a day when I'm training as I need them as fuel. If you're not exercising, you don't need to load up on carbohydrates. And I'll aim to go for good carbs, like porridge, which give you a slow release of energy.

(People often think of breakfast cereal as healthy, but it can have a lot of sugar in it.) I rarely eat pasta unless it's a special occasion or I'm having a really big cheat night. It's something you tend to eat a big bowl of with cheese or creamy sauces and that makes it high in calories, so it's not great food if you're trying to lose weight. I don't really eat rice a lot either, because I feel like it bloats me. But I'll always have bread! I'll just eat it once a week – brown or white, just whatever me mam's got in the cupboard – rather than all the time.

As for sugary foods, I'm lucky not to have much of a sweet tooth, as I know sugar can be so addictive for people. You've got to make sure you think of it as a treat, rather than letting it sneak into your life all the time! But I've not cut anything out. You don't have to do that. If you do, then your diet can become very plain and boring – and you'll get fed up of the whole lifestyle. I wouldn't even say give up chocolate. In fact you can have a square of dark chocolate every single night if you want to – that's what I like to do – admittedly it's an aquired taste but persevere, it's worth it. So don't give up chocolate; don't give up anything! It's about having everything in moderation.

Even fat – you need fats in your diet for your body to work properly. If you're having fats, simply think avocados, nuts and – if you like it – oily fish. Not a deep-fried Mars bar! But you don't have to be super-rigid about it. Yes, I will cut the fatty rind off my meat – it makes me feel sick! – but I will happily eat rich, fatty meats like salami, duck, pork and corned beef, if not all the time. And you need fat to cook in. I've switched to coconut oil, which although it has the same number of calories as other oils, it contains a fat called lauric acid that some people think is a healthier type of fat. I got used to the slight coconut flavour after a while.

But thinking about the food groups all the time can get confusing – and boring. That's why I'm sharing all my favourite recipes, which will give you a good, healthy mix of all the stuff you need, as well as some of my favourite healthy swaps…

HEALTHY SWAPS

WATER!

SWAP FIZZY POP FOR

I always aim for two litres a day, but sometimes I can get about three down. Pretty much all I drink is water. Which of course is the best thing you can drink of all – there's no nasties in it, no empty calories, and it's totally free. The thing is, I don't even really like fizzy pop – it doesn't quench me thirst. Holly from *Geordie Shore* says she doesn't like water, which is the craziest thing I've ever heard! If I'm having a cheat meal and I'm hungover, I'll have a McDonald's and a fizzy Fanta though. I won't do a diet drink, I'll go for the real thing. I don't think diet drinks with artificial sweeteners are very good for you. I'd rather have a proper fizzy pop as a treat than the fake versions all the time.

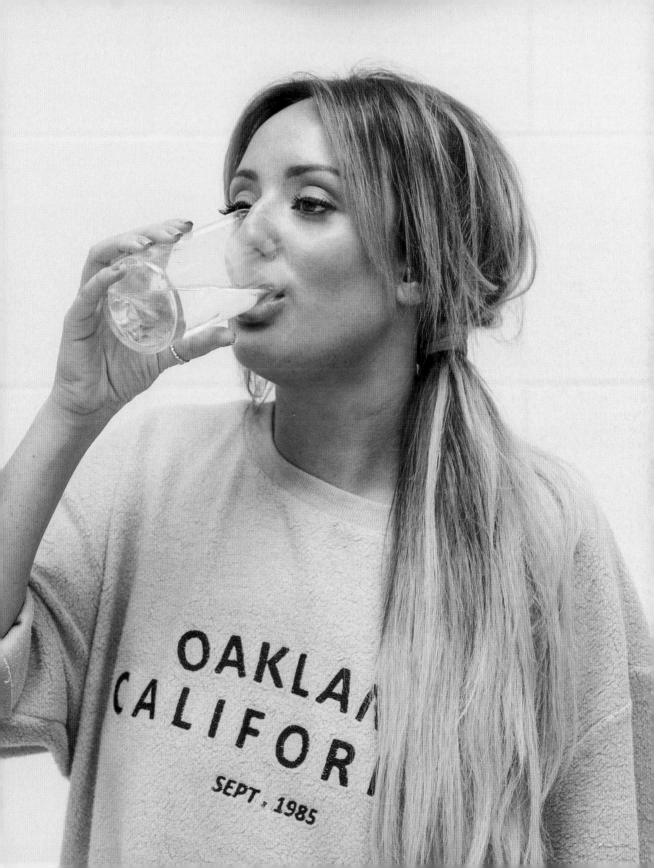

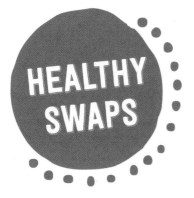

HEALTHY SWAPS

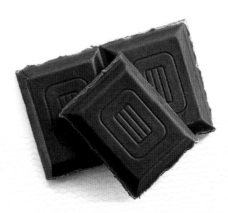

DARK CHOCOLATE

SWAP MILK CHOCOLATE FOR

These days, I eat chocolate with a 90% cocoa content – and I love it. It's an acquired taste, but you get used to it. In fact, I prefer it to Dairy Milk now. It's absolutely gorgeous. It's usually lower in sugar than milk chocolate and because it's got such a punch of flavour I find I don't need to eat so much of it.

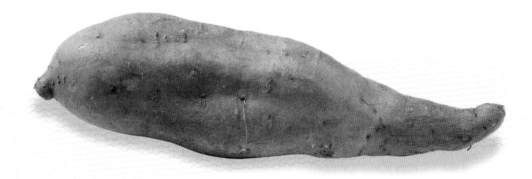

SWEET POTATO

SWAP WHITE POTATO FOR

I'm a big fan of sweet potatoes – as you'll see when you get to the recipe section! Not only do they taste lovely, they are a slow-release carbohydrate which means they give you energy over a longer time. They have more fibre (which doesn't just keep you, ahem, regular – it helps keep you full) than normal potatoes and lots of vitamin A, which is good for your immune system.

HEALTHY SWAPS

GOATS' CHEESE OR HALLOUMI

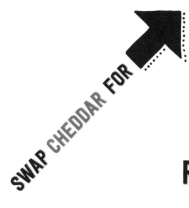

SWAP CHEDDAR FOR

I love cheese, I eat cheese all the time. I'd prefer to have cheese than chocolate. I just go for cheeses that are a bit lower in fat. I love grilled halloumi – it's gorgeous.

RYE OR WHOLEMEAL BREAD

SWAP WHITE BREAD FOR

Both are higher in fibre and more nutritious than the plasticky white stuff. As I said, I have wholemeal (or sometimes white if that's all me mam has in) bread once a week, but I will go for rye bread the rest of the time. I'll eat it just like you would a normal piece of bread: I'll toast it, have it as a sandwich or have it on its own with some peanut butter for a snack.

POPCORN

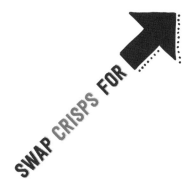

SWAP CRISPS FOR

I love popcorn – it's not as greasy and fatty as crisps. I will have a small bag of salty or sweet popcorn, I won't go for a huge bag of the toffee or caramel, which can be really sugary. Still, I can end up eating a packet a day if I'm not careful! Ideally save it for a bit of a treat, when you're hungry for a snack.

HOT DRINKS WITHOUT THE CRAP THAT WILL MAKE YOU FAT!

SWAP SUGARY TEA AND COFFEE FOR

I don't drink a lot of tea or coffee, but if you do, make sure you're not slurping down loads of sugar with it. If I'm out and about and I need a bit of a boost, I'll go to a coffee shop and I'll have a soy latte. I do love a soy latte – personally, I prefer soy milk to cow's milk. But I drink them quite rarely, every few weeks or so. And remember, some of the fancier takeaway coffees are full of sugary syrups and come covered in those creamy, high-fat toppings. Coffee with a splash of milk is going to be a better choice if you're someone who's always got a paper cup in their hand.

HEALTHY SWAPS

BROWN RICE

SWAP WHITE RICE FOR

If you eat a lot of rice, it's a great idea to eat brown – it's got more fibre and it gives you slower-release energy.

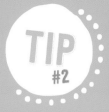

CHARLOTTE'S LIVE FAST LOSE WEIGHT ★TIP★

Got a sweet tooth? A lot of people think going for brown sugar is better than white. Newsflash! One is not healthier than the other. They both come from the same sugar cane, they're just processed slightly differently – and neither of them is going to do you any good. I'm lucky not to have a sweet tooth, but I know sugar can be so addictive for people. If you're reaching for something unhealthy, sometimes it's easier just to say no to start with, rather than aiming to have just the one sweet or biscuit – and then finding you've scoffed the whole packet. Try to save your sugary foods for your cheat meals (more on those later…).

MY DAILY ROUTINE

What I eat does change a bit depending on what I'm up to, and that's fine. At home, it's really quite easy to be healthy. I do 'fasted cardio', which sounds impressive, but just means that in the morning I do my workout before I eat. It's great, because you're burning your fat stores instead of the food you've just eaten. Then, when I get back home I'll have a healthy breakfast. It could be porridge, protein pancakes or, more often than not, eggs. Sometimes I'll have them with tomatoes, mushrooms, a bit of turkey bacon – which is leaner than normal bacon. I call this my 'Healthy fry-up' and you can see the recipe on page 98. Maybe once a week I'll have my eggs with toast. I think having a good breakfast is really important – it will give you energy and set you up for the whole day. That's why I've shared lots of breakfast ideas in the recipe section of the book.

After breakfast I will take Baby, my little dog, out for a walk. I love spending time with Baby and it's always good to be active throughout the whole of the day. (I live with me mam and dad so they look after her when I'm away. Which is annoying, because I feel like she bonds with them more than me. Watch it, Baby!).

I cook all my own meals each day. Before I started this lifestyle, I never really tried to cook because I was always ordering takeaways. I knew I could cook a really good fry-up, but that was it. These days, I tend to eat something coldish for my lunch – one of my salads (like my 'Chicken salad with a bit of everything', or 'Salmon and pesto salad') or soup. For dinner I'll have something nice and hot, like my 'Healthy meatballs with pepper sauce' or the 'Piri piri chicken with sweet roast potatoes'. So tasty.

If I know I'm going to be out and about I sometimes prep my food in advance. When I do, I simply cook the sort of food I normally eat the night before and box it all up. I might make up enough for two so I can get a couple of boxes out of it: chicken salad, veggie stew or my cottage pie. If I have got a microwave handy when I'm away I might heat it up. And I will pack some hard-boiled eggs, little boxes of nuts, yoghurt and fruit, too, to snack on.

If I'm away for longer than a couple of days there's not much point in prepping, though, because I can't always keep the food fresh when I'm in a hotel. That's why, when I'm on the road for work, I live out of shops like Pret A Manger. It's perfect – it's my second home. I can get hard-boiled eggs, healthy salads, porridge – lots of the stuff I'd eat at home. In fact, when I'm on the road Pret's pretty much the only place I eat. If I'm near one I just go in and out all day for my meals. (When I'm on the road, I find I don't really snack because I'm so busy.)

Of course I try to avoid places where there are no healthy options, but sometimes there really is nothing else to eat. In that case, I go for what seems to be the best choice. Sometimes I even adapt what's on offer – I'm not embarrassed to do that at all. If you're at a service station and you're starving and you just have to have a sausage roll, take all the pastry off and just eat the meat in the middle! It's not the best – it's processed meat – but it's a better option than the greasy pastry. In the same way, there's often no healthy option when you're on a plane. So recently when I was flying back from holiday I ordered the chicken pasta – I just ate the chicken and avoided the pasta.

You can see clearly I'm not someone who's sticking to a really strict routine. I do always eat breakfast – it's your fuel for the day and you burn it off just doing normal, everyday things if you have an active day. But I'm not setting any inflexible rules about when you've got to eat. I'm happy to have three meals a day and I prefer not to snack in between. If I do, I find I can over indulge, even with healthy stuff. But if I need to – if I'm starving! – I will have a snack, so I list some of my favourite healthy options on page 44.

I do think sleep's important when you're eating healthily and exercising. It means I'm not tired and grumpy when I'm working out, and I'm less likely to be reaching for an unhealthy snack because I'm desperate for an energy pick-me-up. I mostly get eight hours when I'm not filming. (And sometimes a bit more – I do like a nap in the afternoon if I've had a big training session in the morning! I find when I wake up from a nap, though, I'm the hungriest I ever get. A mystery of life!)

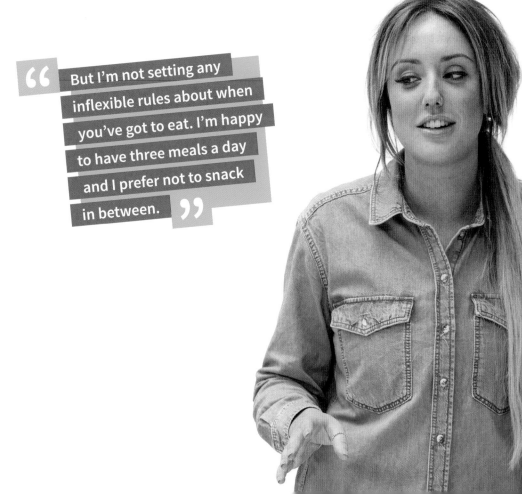

" But I'm not setting any inflexible rules about when you've got to eat. I'm happy to have three meals a day and I prefer not to snack in between. "

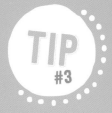
TIP #3

CHARLOTTE'S LIVE FAST LOSE WEIGHT ★TIP★

You hear a lot about portion size – but how are you supposed to know when just right turns into too much? Of course, you've got to listen to your body and think about if you're feeling satisfied… or if you're about to get too stuffed. But that can take a bit of practice as you get used to eating healthily. So here's my dead simple way of getting on board with sensible portions. Instead of a big plate, I will put all of my food on a little one. It's a great trick because it means you're choosing smaller portions and not over eating – but you don't even notice it! And remember to have a big glass of water a bit before your meal, to make sure you're eating because you're actually hungry, not just thirsty (yes, your body can get these confused. Well, no one said it was Albert Einstein…).

WHY I HATE CALORIE-COUNTING

I never was someone to faff about with food. I know some people are full of rules, like: eat just the egg whites and avoid the yolks, because the yolks have more fat and calories than the whites. Don't bother! You've got to make this workable for you. If you've got a healthy lifestyle and you're exercising, there's no need to worry about egg yolks.

In the same way, I don't really calorie-count. I know roughly what's in each of my meals, just as a guesstimate, but I don't sit and work out what each meal represents. For me, a healthy calorie consumption would probably be between 1,200 and 1,500 calories per day, but I'm not going to try and track every little thing I'm eating. Again, who can really be bothered to do that long term? Very rarely, I will use a fitness app just to see how many calories are in my food – sometimes you don't realise exactly. Say if I've been very healthy in terms of what foods I've been eating, but I've eaten a lot, I might think, 'I wonder, how many calories I've actually eaten today?' So I'll look, just out of curiosity.

Don't get too obsessed about calorie-counting though. Sometimes the healthiest of foods can contain a lot of calories, but it doesn't matter. For example, nuts are very high in calories, but you're not eating badly by eating a few protein-rich nuts. Hummus, too, has a lot of calories and a lot of fat – but it's good fat that your body needs. Even a piece of chicken breast is about 300 calories. But you can't count that as being 'bad' – it's protein and you need it. The other day I had a Nando's salad which, I discovered, was quite calorific because it was packed with avocado and nuts – good foods full of nutrients that your body needs. So I didn't look at it and think, 'I'm going to stop eating this.' I didn't change. The key is just moderation.

GIMME A NIBBLE

As I said, it's great to aim for three proper meals a day and stay out of the fridge in between. But we're only human! There are times when all you want to do is snack on something. You'll have your meal and that's fine, but in between you've got your go-to things you just want to grab and have a little taste of. So you might as well make sure they're good for you. I wasn't a big biscuit or sweet fan in the first place, but I started snacking on healthy savoury stuff (instead of grabbing some junk food!).

I never used to like olives, but I'd see Sophie from *Geordie Shore* eating them all the time, and I got curious. They're an acquired taste, but now I love them. They're packed with fibre, vitamin E – good for your skin – and healthy fats. Mmm, olives.

Or I might have hummus and carrots, or a little pack of prawns or cockles. I love cockles. You can buy pickled cockles in a jar, drain them out and just pick at them. They're full of protein and they're bloody gorgeous. You can get them in the supermarket… or the chip shop! Pickled onions, too, are a great snack if you like the taste – full of flavour and nothing bad in them.

Nuts are sneaky. They're great for you, but completely addictive. At one point I had to stop eating nuts because I was eating too many! So here's my little trick to getting the right portion of nuts. Always make sure it's a small handful – sometimes I pile it a little too high so it's spilling off my hand – but no more than a handful. And if you've had your handful, and you want to go back for more? Slap yourself in the face with the hand that just ate the nuts! Because you shouldn't. That's when you start eating too many.

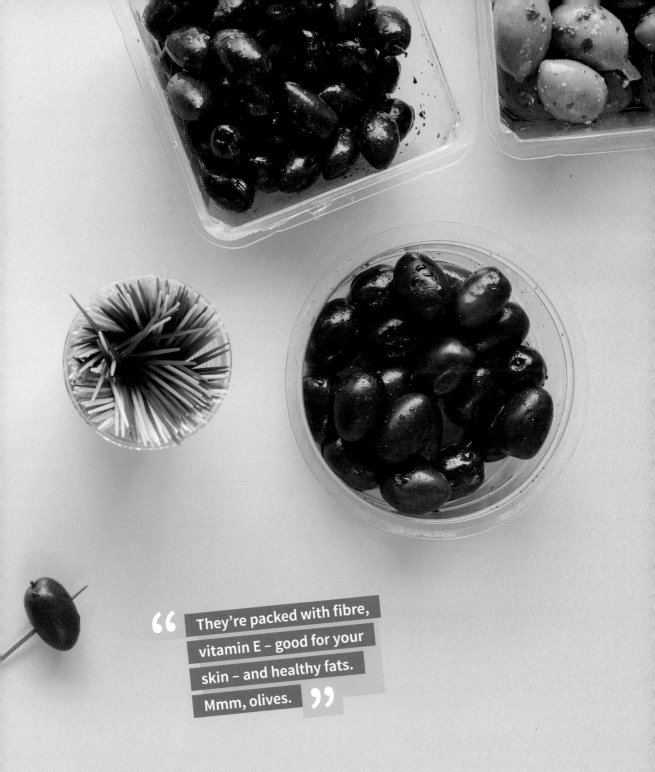

"They're packed with fibre, vitamin E – good for your skin – and healthy fats. Mmm, olives."

Sometimes I snack on plain Greek yoghurt – the 0% fat version – as it's got more protein than other types of yoghurt. You can have it with a sprinkle of nuts, some fruit or a little drizzle of honey. But you know what I really like? Jelly. I'll buy those little ready-made pots if I'm out and about, in orange, blackberry, strawberry. As a little treat. Which leads me neatly to…

CHEATS AND TREATS

When I was losing the weight, eating well and exercising, I'd always look forward to my cheat night when I'd eat whatever I felt like. I thought of it as my reward for being good the rest of the time! These days, if I'm trying to lose a bit of weight, I aim for one cheat night a week and really look forward to it. If I'm where I want to be, I might have two a week.

But I've never been perfect about it. At the very beginning of all this, I was having about three cheat nights a week! Yes, I was eating well for the rest of the time and I was exercising. But three evenings out of each week I'd eat whatever I fancied. And every so often – I'm talking every few months, not every few weeks – I just went all-out with a cheat day. I'd have a cheat breakfast, cheat lunch, cheat snacks. And it was always, always, always McDonald's; I'm obsessed with McDonald's.

And still I saw the changes; still the weight was coming off. That's one of the encouraging things about getting started. Because, at first – at least, this is what I found and I know other people have had similar experiences – when you're at your biggest, it feels as if the weight drops off almost no matter what. At the slightest change in your lifestyle, it comes off! It's like your body's so ready to lose it. It's when you're further down the line, closer to your goal weight, that you need to make bigger changes. I still slip up though. But these days, I tell

CHARLOTTE'S
CHEAT DAY

Breakfast

A fry-up.

Or a McDonald's breakfast.

Lunch

A Big Mac Meal with fizzy Fanta.

A Double Cheeseburger.

(I don't eat the bread – well, I might have one half of the bun, but not all of it.)

Six Chicken Nuggets and two Sour Cream Dips.

This is, without fail, my McDonald's order. I have to have it.

Snacks and sweet treats. Crisps galore.

Although I don't have much of a sweet tooth, I like a sticky toffee pudding.

And cupcakes.

I cannot say no to a cupcake. It's doesn't matter what flavour, any cupcake, I will have them all.

Dinner

By this time, I'd be quite full – because I'd eaten a load of shit! And normally cheat days are on hangover days, so I'd probably be lying in bed watching *The Vampire Diaries* and couldn't even be bothered to go downstairs.

myself, 'Charlotte, why are you beating yourself up about it? You slipped up all the way through the process. But you lost two and a half stone. One day doesn't make a difference.'

I mean, I went wrong so many times! I was on *Geordie Shore*, still drinking loads, having McDonald's. I remember one day, while I was on a break from the show, I'd been doing really well with my healthy diet and I'd gone to the gym. Then me mam texted me, saying, 'Nathaniel [that's my brother] has been really good at school and I want to give him a treat. Can you get a chicken nugget Happy Meal and bring it home with you on the way back?' I thought, 'Right, okay.' I went to get his Happy Meal – and ended up buying myself a twenty-nugget share box! I ate ten nuggets straightaway: 'Oh, if only I didn't have to go to McDonald's, man!'

But it didn't change anything. I beat myself up about it and for what reason? None. Did I put two stone back on? No. Everyone is going to have their little cheats. My friends will say we're going out for a meal, and maybe some people would think I should really say, 'Oh girls, I'm trying to be good.' Instead, I say, 'Yeah, I'll come.' And sometimes I'll end up eating all the food off their plates…

BEWARE THE 'SOD IT' SPIRAL

That brings me to my biggest tip of all for you, which I tell myself all the time, ever since I've started being healthier: don't EVER feel like you've let yourself down or that you've failed. Because the second that you think that, that's it. From then on you start knocking down everything you're doing. Say you've had a little unplanned cheat, had a packet of crisps, and you think, 'Right, I've failed.' And because you think of yourself as a failure, you decide: 'Well, I might as well just eat badly for the rest of the day now.' And that day turns into another, and another, and then a whole week's gone and you've carried on eating badly through it all.

★

CHARLOTTE'S
WORDS OF WISDOM

TO WEIGH OR NOT TO WEIGH?

Some people find monitoring their weight really motivating, and that checking it every day really works for them. I find that weighing meself all the time can be quite demotivating so I try not to jump on the scales too often. I prefer to weigh meself every couple of weeks so that each time I see a bigger change. I always make sure I do it first thing in the morning when my stomach is empty as then I can see my actual body weight. Remember, fluctuations can be caused by lots of things like the time of the month, stress, and even when you last went to the loo. You could just be carrying round a mammoth poo! But to be honest, I don't worry too much about weight, I prefer to think about how I feel and how my clothes are fitting and how much energy I've got.

When I was bigger, I'd make this same mistake all the time. If I was at a photo shoot, where they usually put out a buffet, I'd pick up a piece of bread, smother it in peanut butter or chocolate spread, eat it and then I'd think, 'Oh no, what have I done?' Inevitably, I'd go through that process of telling myself, 'I've been bad.' But you can't beat yourself up about a treat. I don't think anyone needs to eat perfectly every single minute of the day. So nowadays, I still might have some bread and spread. But the trap I try to avoid is turning that one indulgence into something much bigger – not just a cheat treat, but a cheat week.

You've just got to avoid that spiralling: 'That's it now. I've been bad. I might as well keeping eating bad.' Even now, I catch myself at it. The other week, when I was on holiday in Cape Verde, I was trying to be really healthy and I had an ice cream. 'Damn,' I thought. 'That's it now. I failed. I might as well eat rubbish now for the rest of the week.' And you beat yourself up about it – and there is NO POINT. Imagine an obese person going on a diet for one day and eating badly for the rest of the week. It's not going to make a difference, is it? In the same way, if you're eating really well for a whole week and have one bad day, it isn't going to make a difference. So the second you start thinking in that way, you've got to catch yourself and ask: 'Well, have I failed? This isn't going to make a difference so long as I eat well for the rest of the week. It's not failure, it's being a human being!'

Have your treat, allow it, enjoy it and don't beat yourself up about it.

Then…

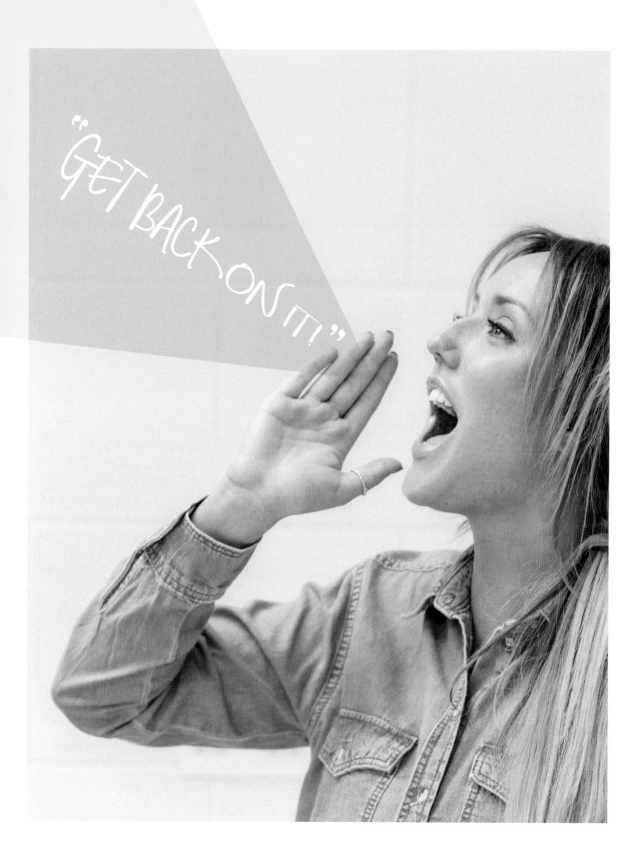

"GET BACK ON IT!"

MIND THE TRAP

The shame spiral's not the only mindset you've got to avoid. Here are a few more unhelpful thoughts…

It's too expensive for me to eat healthily
Is it though? You can buy a whole chicken for under a fiver. I get all my fruit and veg from Aldi, the budget supermarket. So that's just a massive excuse! None of the recipes in this book relies on pricey ingredients – it's all just easy-to-find, everyday stuff.

I've no time to cook
That's not important at all. Being healthy isn't complicated, you don't have to sit down and make yourself a meal. I'm on the road all the time and you can even get healthy food on the go. Here's one of my favourite lazy meals: I go to a supermarket, I get a pack of cooked chicken pieces, a pack of salad and a little pot of hummus (one of the those mini ones you get in a pack of three) – and mix it all together. Done!

But let's be honest, most people have got fifteen to twenty minutes in the day to cook something quick. So, when you do feel like cooking, then all my recipes in this book are really easy to make – often just putting together nice, tasty ingredients that you probably have in already!

I don't know about all this healthy eating lark – protein powders and chia seeds scare me!
Fine. I'm not that experimental person who's all, 'Let's put loads of mysterious seeds and spices in our foods.' I'm a real person who needs to do something that's easily available to me, not complicated at all. My recipes are straightforward and simple – but still taste great.

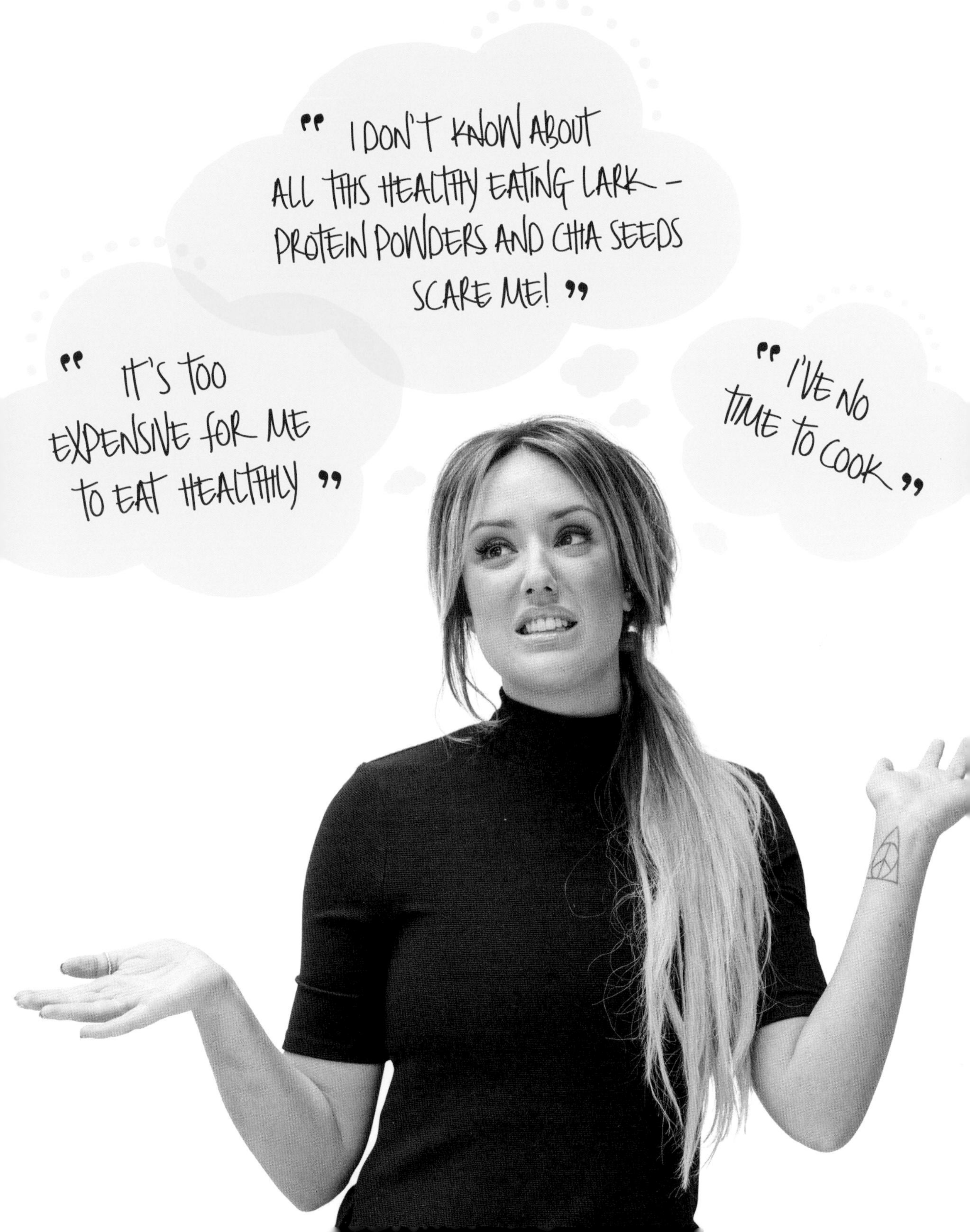
"I DON'T KNOW ABOUT ALL THIS HEALTHY EATING LARK – PROTEIN POWDERS AND CHIA SEEDS SCARE ME!"
"IT'S TOO EXPENSIVE FOR ME TO EAT HEALTHILY"
"I'VE NO TIME TO COOK"

CHARLOTTE'S WORDS OF WISDOM

WHY YOU SHOULDN'T TURN CHRISTMAS INTO A CHEAT MONTH

I remember thinking one December, 'Oh it's Christmas soon, I'm going to go all-out.' And then I thought, 'Why?' It's like saying, 'My birthday's in May, so I'm going to have a blow-out every day that month.' Those other days aren't special. I normally go out on Christmas Eve with my friends – it's a tradition. We'll get absolutely steaming drunk and wake up with the worst hangovers ever. On Christmas Day, I'll open my selection box and eat it all for breakfast! Then it's all the family round for a big lovely roast. And Boxing Day is much the same. So Christmas Eve, Christmas Day and Boxing Day are all pig-out days for me. And if you've been good for the whole of that month – if you've been exercising, if you've been eating well – three days are not going to make a difference in the slightest! But remember: it's just three days. You don't have to spend the rest of the month the same way.

YOU GOTTA WORK

As I said, people always ask me what I eat – but that's not the whole story. If it were, then a lot more people would be strutting around looking amazing! But being fit and having a good body is about working hard for it – and, yes, that includes exercise. While eating healthily is great – you will lose weight, it's perfect for that – if you want to feel and look your absolute best, to get toned as well as slim, you need to pull your finger out. These days I never go too long without some kind of workout. And even when I'm in the *Geordie Shore* house, I exercise – at least three sessions a week.

Don't feel you have to be great at your workout from the start, or anything like that. The other day, I fell off the step at one of my training classes in front of everyone – that was a bit awkward. But who cares? It was hilarious. At the moment, I train five times a week, but at other times I'll be doing fewer sessions – it depends what I've got going on. You always need at least one rest day a week for your body to recover. They actually help you lose weight – your muscles repair and rebuild themselves after all that exercise and, mentally, you get a break so you don't get tired and fed up with the whole thing.

Three is the magic number! Try to exercise at least three times a week. It's a healthy amount, it's not overexerting yourself and it's quite manageable for people with busy lifestyles. But if you've got the time, go for four. Maybe even five, and have the weekend off! It could be my DVD, cardio, weights – whatever works for you. So long as you're doing something.

If I can do it, you can too. Everyone makes excuses, don't they? Sometimes I can say to myself, 'Oh, I've been good all week. I don't need to do a workout.' I'm always thinking, 'Oh I'll just do it tomorrow.' Everyone does that with their diet too: 'I'll start again tomorrow.' You have to tell yourself, 'NO! Do it right now.' That exact second you start thinking about putting it off? Get it out of the way. This is where my DVD routines are so good because they're short three-minute blitzes. A twenty-minute workout is what all the experts recommend, and let's face it, that's just a few combinations from the DVD. And if three minutes is all you can manage, then three minutes are better than no minutes.

And everyone has those days when they've got no energy and they're dragging themselves around. I have them a lot. You could be doing cardio or a run on the treadmill, and after five minutes, you think, 'I've got to turn this down a bit, I need to walk for a bit.' Well so what? You're still walking! You're still doing something. I find I perform better in the afternoons. In the mornings, I will moan all the way through. Then later my trainer will tell me, 'What the hell, you're like a different person!' Still, there's no such thing as a bad workout, so long as you've done one. (There are loads of inspirational quotes on the wall at my gym. Sometimes they rub off!) Being active is ten times better than lying in bed or sitting on the settee. The simple fact that you've done a workout is great. You've actually exercised.

★

CHARLOTTE'S
WORDS OF WISDOM

WHY YOU SHOULD
WORK OUT ON HOLIDAY

On holiday, you're faced with temptation every minute. There are buffets, there are ice cream parlours, there are cocktails, there are fishbowls – there's temptation everywhere. And you want to be able to enjoy yourself! So that's why exercise is the best tip that I can give to anyone who doesn't want to come home half a stone heavier. You only have to do it once a day – for even just half an hour if you want to – and then that's it, you relax. Trying to think about eating healthily every second of the day is so much harder than trying to work out for half an hour every day. So, my advice is to eat a healthy breakfast (even at a buffet you can make good choices, like boiled eggs, slices of ham, fruit) and a healthy lunch. Indulge in the night-time – maybe have a nice snack too – but try and do at least a half-hour workout each day. You don't need a gym to work out on holiday, but if your hotel does have one that's a bonus. When I'm away I like to do short circuits in the morning, or if I'm with a boyfriend I like to have loads of sex and count that as a workout too!

LIVING MY LIFE

So now you've got the basics down. I know what you're thinking: when am I going to see results?

First of all, you need to be clear on what results you want. I found it helpful to have a goal, not just a vague idea that I was going to 'get skinny'.

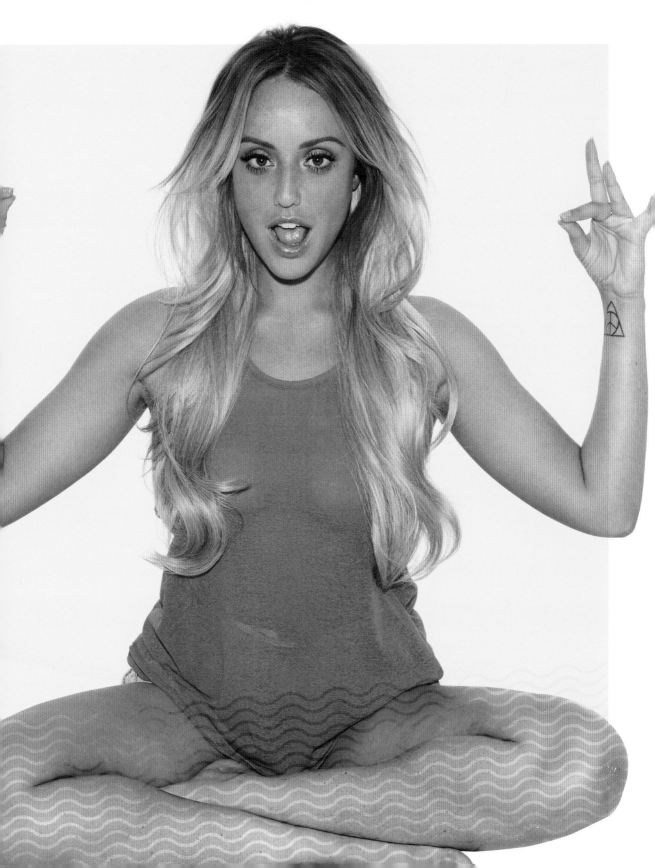

What I did was, I worked out what was a healthy weight for my size and that's what I aimed for – I researched it on the internet and set out a target weight with my trainer. (I realise not everyone has a trainer! But there are lots of tools online on how to work out a sensible weight for your height and build if you're really not sure, or you could ask your GP or a dietician.) Once I'd started, I monitored my weight and my measurements, and just kept track of how I fit in my clothes.

Mind you, I don't use scales much now I've lost the weight. What I'm looking at these days is dropping my body fat and gaining more muscle – which is denser and more compact than fat so your weight may go up as you lay down more tight muscle mass. But even if I am going up in weight I look exactly the same – if not better – because I'm toning up. I'm doing it by using weights and doing resistance training, and eating a bit more protein, which is great for building muscle. A lot of people think working out is all about cardio but it's not – weights and resistance training are brilliant, because the more muscle you have the more calories you burn. So while it's fine to track how you're changing on the scales, don't get obsessed by it. It's not the be-all and end-all.

In fact, these days I see nine stone – around a size six to eight on my frame – as my healthy weight. That's a little bit heavier than my lowest, when I went down to eight stone nine while I was on a big break from *Geordie Shore* and could be really dedicated to the gym and eating well. Now, because I'm currently in and out of *Geordie Shore* – where you live that intense party lifestyle – I'm always fluctuating, and I tend to stick at nine. When I next go back into the house I'm going to take my scales, so I can keep an eye on where I am. But like I've said, if I'm eating healthily I won't weigh meself all the time, only every couple of weeks or so. If you know you're feeling good and looking good, what's the point?

★

CHARLOTTE'S
WORDS OF WISDOM

NO GYM?
NO EXCUSE!

Honestly, you don't need a gym to do exercise. We've got a tiny little gym with a few weights in the *Geordie Shore* house, and I'll do weights in there once a week. But on another day, I'll do my DVD in the sitting room. I won't just run through all the sections from start to finish – I might start from the end and work backwards! I change it up every time. And then on another day, I'll do circuits in the back garden incorporating moves from my DVD. So, I'll do squat jumps on the bench, I'll do tricep dips on the little wooden chair, then I'll do burpees*. Then I'll move inside the house to sprint up and down the stairs. Use the furniture, be imaginative! Because I find exercise does get boring I need to be constantly changing it up. If I don't, I get bored and think, 'I can't be bothered to do this again!' Nathan's my workout buddy in the house, which spurs me on. There've been a couple of times where he hasn't joined in, but I think, 'Right, just because Nathan's not doing it, doesn't mean I'm not going to do it.' I'll feel better that I've got up and done it on my own.

★ If you've never done them, have a look online, but basically you squat with your hands on the ground, kick your feet back so you're in a push-up position, do a push-up, get back into a squat, then jump straight up with your hands in the air... and start it all over again. They're killer!

THE WEIGHT-LOSS WAIT

If you're looking at the scales you'll soon start to see the numbers dropping, but in terms of spotting physical changes it will take a bit longer. I reckon I started to notice them at about four weeks. And then I felt like there were loads of times when the weight just didn't come off – when my body didn't change. That's really common. But *don't stress about it*. Your weight loss is not going to be the same every week, or even every month. And that's really okay. You're not a machine.

Don't worry either if you feel like no one's noticed you're changing. When I first began trying to lose weight I didn't want to tell that many people – because I didn't know if I was going to do it or if I was going to fail. I *did* do it and you can do it too. Trust me! But I had to tell them in the end. Some of that was practical. One of my bad habits, I knew, was eating slices of corned beef straight out of the fridge. I had to ask me mam to stop buying it! So, me best friends knew, me mam, me dad, me agent – but I didn't tell anyone from *Geordie Shore*. I was scared in case I didn't manage to lose the weight and then they'd be able to say to me: 'You've been talking the talk, but you didn't do it.' I had to tell them after a while, because they found out about the exercise DVD I was making! Still, I didn't feel like anyone noticed me changing. The 'Oh, you're losing weight' comments only started when I'd lost quite a considerable amount – about a stone and a half. Just remember: everybody will notice in the end!

But in case you need a little motivation before then, I feel like it's time for another poem…

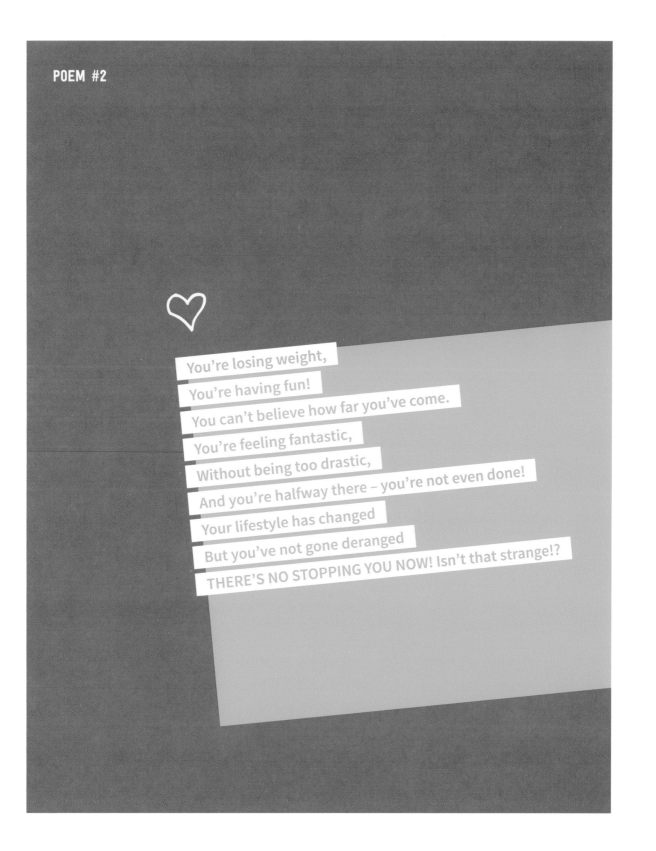

You're losing weight,

You're having fun!

You can't believe how far you've come.

You're feeling fantastic,

Without being too drastic,

And you're halfway there – you're not even done!

Your lifestyle has changed

But you've not gone deranged

THERE'S NO STOPPING YOU NOW! Isn't that strange!?

And now for the best bit – I'm going to tell you how you can still have an amazing time living this lifestyle! Here's my main rule… wait for it…

CHARLOTTE'S #1 RULE

GO OUT AS MUCH AS YOU WANT!

JUST MAKE SURE…
YOU EAT WELL
AND ARE EXERCISING.

WILD NIGHTS AND RICE CAKES

My job is being on *Geordie Shore*, where I go out every night for six weeks. When I'm not in the show's house, I don't go mad every night, but I will go out for a big night once a week or once a fortnight. Now, we all know booze is just empty calories. So, if I know that I'm going to have a night out at the weekend (so it's planned, obviously; if it's a random night out it goes to pot), I'll be good all week. I want to look great in whatever I'm wearing. And then during that day, I will try to be spot on with what I eat because I know that I'm going to be having a lot of calories that night. You balance it out. Anyway, if I'm excited about an evening I'm not thinking about food as much as usual anyway – I'm busy getting prepared! I will also train the day I'm going to go out if I have time.

Say, the other day, when I was out and about for work, I had figs for breakfast – I love figs – and then a supermarket chicken salad for lunch. In the evening, there was food at the event, so I had one of the burgers – without the bun – and some salad. I still had three meals but I made absolutely sure they were dead on, because I knew I'd be making up for it with the drink in terms of calories. And then at the end of the night, when I had the drunken hunger, I had a big packet of rice cakes, which was another healthy option. But I'm not going to lie: that's only because the kebab shop wasn't open!

In all honesty, I don't hold meself back in terms of drinking because I'm on *Geordie Shore*, a show all about going wild and getting mortal. Drink is a big part of my life when we're filming. On the show there are no limitations and we go out every night. I go hell for leather; I treat it as if it's a holiday. It's not a place where you can stop and worry about anything, because you haven't got time. And I drink everything in there: vodka and soda, gin and tonic, rum and Coke, white wine. This is the thing with me: the diet doesn't take control of my

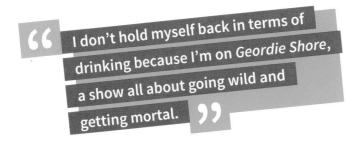

" I don't hold myself back in terms of drinking because I'm on *Geordie Shore*, a show all about going wild and getting mortal. "

life. I will live my life – I can't go through it being the same way the whole time. Everyone is going to fluctuate in weight. I'm a human being – not a robot – and I've managed to fix things this way so I'll stick to it. As long as I'm maintaining a healthy lifestyle and diet most of the time, that's all I care about.

Ooh, the morning after, this is the testing time. This is when you need to *really* try and be healthy, and it's so hard. What I do is I have a cheat meal, but I don't make it a cheat day. So, you could go to McDonald's in the morning and have a breakfast, or have a bacon sarnie, but for the rest of the day, try to eat well. Or, I might have a cheat meal later, and start the day with a bowl of porridge: lots of milk, some honey or some nuts. It's got healthy carbs and good fats. Porridge keeps you feeling full – it's more substantial than a piece of fruit which would leave you starving afterwards – and it will keep you ticking over for the rest of the day.

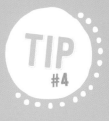

CHARLOTTE'S LIVE FAST LOSE WEIGHT ★TIP★

We all know that alcohol's not good for you and, if you're really, really good you'll stick to soft drinks. I'm not that good at being good! On a night out, I normally drink vodka and water, instead of a traditional mixer. I find I don't get much of a hangover the next day – I can't say for sure, but I wonder if that's because so much of a hangover is dehydration and all that water helps with that. Plus, vodka and any mixer is a lower-calorie option. I sometimes have some lemon, but normally I just have ice.

CHARLOTTE'S
WORDS OF WISDOM

WORKING OUT ON A HANGOVER

I do this all the time in the *Geordie Shore* house. Nearly every morning I'm hungover, but that's no excuse not to do it. What, you've got a bit of a hangover, a bit of a sore head? Have a good breakfast. Get up and get out. Sweat it out. You'll feel so much better. I don't have any special gentle hangover routine, if I'm going to exercise, I'll go all-in – do my DVD, head to the gym, whatever – hungover or not.

DRESSED TO KILL

There's a really big plus to a night out or a big event when you're getting healthy and fit: the clothes. I've started to dress so differently compared to when I was first getting healthy – because obviously I feel a lot better now.

You can see that in my clothing range, which I began when I was bigger. If you look at the first range, it used to be all baggy stuff – baggy tops, baggy skirts, baggy dresses. You wouldn't see a tight thing in there, it was like I wanted to hide myself away a bit, or at least the parts of me I wasn't so keen on. Now my line, Nostalgia, is all cut-out bits, deep V-necks, lovely little dresses and tiny outfits – I've even been out at night in just a Guns N' Roses leotard and boots! (Well, I did wear a shirt over it.) It's almost like I'd rather walk around naked! And yes, sometimes, I do when I've had a lot to drink in the *Geordie Shore* house…

So my style changed a lot.

But, more importantly, how I felt about myself changed. On *Geordie Shore*, us girls are always running out of outfits because we're going out all the time. You end up wearing anything. Now I'm feeling better about myself and more confident in how I look, I don't mind just shoving anything on. There's no worrying and fretting about it. Which is a really nice way to be.

And dressing well's not confined to a night out either. I used to wear awful things to the gym at the start. I looked like an absolute tramp – I'd be in my boyfriend's shorts and a big top of his. Now that I feel great, I love getting new gym clothes and being girly with it. I tend not to be that adventurous with me normal fashion, so I do go a bit out there with me gym clothes. I'm very outrageous. Normally I don't like to wear a lot of bright colours, but at the gym I look like

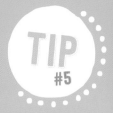

CHARLOTTE'S LIVE FAST LOSE WEIGHT ★TIP★

If I've got an event where I really want to look good, I avoid bread because I find gluten – the proteins found in wheat – makes me bloat like mad. But you might be lucky. I know Holly eats a lot of gluten and she doesn't feel any effects at all. Bitch!

I'm going to a rave, with the amount of neon I'm in. You don't need to spend a bomb. I just look on the high street and buy anything that's nice.

And you know what? I do feel a lot better if I go to the gym in kit I like. I'll be thinking, 'Ooh God, I look quite good.' And that will push me on to do even better 'I'm feeling good, I'll push this workout really hard.' I never wear make-up to the gym unless I've been in the green-screen filming room for *Geordie Shore*, though. Then, I might run straight to the gym afterwards and get there with my show make-up on.

If I'm doing my DVD by meself at home, I will be a bit more relaxed about what I'm wearing – there's not really anyone to show off to and I don't want to get my nice gym kit sweaty in my sitting room! At home I like to wear a baggy top to train and some leggings – that's what I feel comfortable in and is what I always used to the wear to the gym too when I first started exercising and didn't want it all hanging out.

I know a lot of people who go to the gym just in sports bras, but even now I wouldn't do that because exercising doesn't put you in the most flattering positions. I don't want to be looking down at my body and thinking, 'Oh I don't want to be in this position.' But if you do want to exercise in a little bra top, go for it! The thing is to just dress the best way to make you put in the maximum effort for your workout. You don't want to dress stupidly and then have to cut your session short because you feel a bit uncomfortable that your rolls are hanging out, or your sports bra is digging in too tight and that's all you've brought with you. Dress so you're ready to work out hard.

★

CHARLOTTE'S
WORDS OF WISDOM

TINY LITTLE
GYM SHORTS

Steer clear. I mean, with most of my movements in my DVD, you could get a really bad camel toe, or a flap could hang out or something! You could have a big mishap with little shorts. Consider yourself warned.

FRIENDS AND FRENEMIES

So… that's *you* sorted. There's just the question of other people…

In the *Geordie Shore* house, I'm not the only one who's lost weight and toned up – and that's not a coincidence. Vicky Pattison was the first – she did a great job and I think we all looked at her and thought, 'Wow, Vicky looks amazing.' Holly and Sophie, meanwhile, lost weight slowly over the years we were doing the show together. And then I did it. Now we really can say we all feel great for it and we look great! You can really take inspiration from the people around you, and spur each other on.

Of course it can work the other way too! 'Go on, have one, I will.' I'm really guilty of all that. One time I was in the *Geordie Shore* house and spied a big bag of Millie's Cookies. Gary had just bought them and they were still lovely and warm. 'Come on, let's all do it,' I said to the girls. Because if feels so much better if you all do it! And we had about three cookies each. But as I say, if you want to, do it. It's not BAD. Just get back on it later. I remember going on the scales that week – this was when I still weighed meself – and it hadn't affected us at all! Because it was three cookies, one day. The rest of the week I'd been perfectly fine. I'd beaten meself up about it all week – 'I've put weight on!' – and it hadn't made any difference. (It affected Gary though: he was so angry we'd polished off his cookies. He probably would have eaten them all himself, too.)

I've found though – and I hope you will too – that my willpower's got stronger as I've gone on. The other day, I was filming *Geordie Shore* and everyone – all the cast and all the crew – got fish and chips, except me. I wanted to have a healthier day. I'm not a stubborn personality, I'm a pushover, and I'm easily led as well. Even when I'm planning to stay in, if everyone's telling me, 'Come out come out,' I'm all, 'OK, let's go!' But I've kept up my lifestyle while living the same life I led before, still going out every night and drinking a lot and being on *Geordie Shore* – in fact, being on the show and keeping up with my healthy lifestyle has been the hardest part.

My friendships didn't change when I lost weight, but I know sometimes you might find the people close to you don't react how you want. I remember once, all us *Geordie Shore* lot came back from Ibiza and the rest of the cast were in Greggs, getting pasties. 'Ah, I don't want one and me mam's waiting,' I said. 'I've already been bad on the flight.' That didn't go down too well. 'God, Charlotte, don't get on to us, you used to be like this at one point!' I wasn't having a go at them at all. You just have to see it as motivational when you get comments like that – it shows how much you've changed.

And if people go further, and actually make proper digs at you? Think of it as a good thing – they've noticed it and they're feeling threatened – it means you're doing well. Then go find some nicer friends! I'm lucky, no one I know ever faced that situation. There are three other people I know well who've lost weight – Vicky, Holly and Sophie – and we were all dead supportive of each other. I think it's really important to have that backing from your friends and family. Getting the odd compliment now and then, people recognising the hard work that you've done – it spurs you on.

"IF ME MATES CAN DO IT, I CAN DO IT TOO!"

BE THE BEST YOU

While it can be nice to be inspired by other people, you've got to beware of comparing yourself to them. You can't have unrealistic expectations – you've got to think of your own body type. I look at Holly, one of my best friends in *Geordie Shore*, and I think, 'Wow, Holly has got an hourglass figure.' She goes in and out in all the right places. I'm never going to be like that, because that's not my body shape at all. I've got dead long legs, but with that comes a shorter torso – more belly fitting into a smaller space! – so I've got to work really hard to make me stomach look good.

But don't think about the negatives. Ask yourself, 'What do I love best about my body?' I love my legs – I've always loved my legs, I loved my legs when I was bigger as well – and I love my arms. And I didn't say this to myself when I was bigger, but when I look back, what I should have been saying is not, 'Oh, I hate me belly and I look fat,' but, 'I love me legs, I'm happy with me arms, and I like me boobs. If everything else gets better, and I change the rest of meself, I'm just going to love more parts of me.' It's about taking a positive attitude, which will help motivate you to change your lifestyle and get healthy.

I mean, some people are just lucky! I was on *Ex on the Beach* with a girl called Anita, a model, who could eat whatever she wanted and not put on weight. Can you imagine? But you just need to realise what kind of person you are. Are you the 'lucky' one, or have you got to work hard for it? Realistically, most people are going to have to put the effort in. To be honest, I'd rather work hard for it because at least I can be proud of myself. I don't think I'd want to be the lucky person. (Well, I mean I would. I'm not mad. But you'd eat rubbish and you wouldn't actually be healthy.) At least you know you're working hard for it, and you're fit and mentally feeling good. And remember… if you go up against each other in a race or a workout, you're going to be the one who wins, aren't you?!

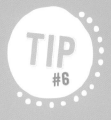

CHARLOTTE'S
LIVE FAST
LOSE WEIGHT
★TIP★

As well as using your social circle, you can use social media as a positive force. I started following Instagram accounts that post really good recipe ideas or motivational quotes. And I do like to take pictures of what I'm eating because it's nice to show off to people that I'm being healthy! But not every meal. Not all the time!

BOYS BOYS BOYS

After I lost weight, boys did find me more attractive. But I didn't really care. I'm not a really sexual, flirty person. I'm more of a person who has a laugh. And a good boyfriend should love you whatever your weight – if you want to change anything, you should do it for yourself and for no one else.

As I write, because I've finished with my ex, Mitch, I haven't yet gone through that stage of a relationship where you can get really comfortable – nights eating pizza in front of the TV, and all that – at the same time as living this lifestyle. And I've yet to get past that stage when you don't really eat in front of the boy you're seeing because you get a bit nervous and excited. So I'm hoping I don't struggle with it! It's not hard to pick a healthy option when you go out to eat, though. And now there are lots more healthy chains that do chicken, salads and other good options – I'll order bunless burgers, corn on the cob, nice salads. The other day I got a chicken burger, no bun, with goats' cheese on top and loads of jalapeños. Gorgeous. Just go for protein and veg, as usual – or the closest you can get to that!

TO INFINITY... AND BEYOND!

Or, what next? Once you've reached your target weight and are feeling good, well done! Give yourself a massive pat on the back. That's from me. Now, you've just got to keep up the good work and you don't have to stress yourself out about trying to lose any more weight. So it's pretty simple – you've just got to stick to what you were doing but you can allow yourself a bit more slack. (I found I could allow myself a lot more treats. Which is all good!)

Remember: strict diets hardly ever work, because at some point you end up eating badly and you think, 'Well, I can't do this anymore. I can't face another egg/apple/cabbage [insert whatever crazy diet you're on]. I've broken the rules and I'm going to give up now. I can't be this strict and carry this on.' But that's not what all of this is about. We're having a life with a good balance of eating healthily, exercising, treating ourselves… and, in my case, getting mortal.

And if you find it all going a bit wrong? Just keep hold of your willpower, stay strong – and get back on it!

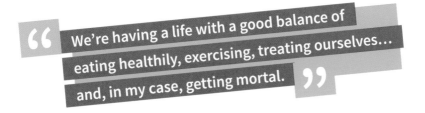

> We're having a life with a good balance of eating healthily, exercising, treating ourselves… and, in my case, getting mortal.

Juice fasts? Maple syrup cleanses? What a load of bullshit! I lost weight and keep it off by working out regularly and eating right – not rabbit food that leaves me starving for a pick-me-up, but by making meself proper, tasty meals (and, yes, some treats!). But don't panic, I'm not about to turn into Nigella. These are quick, dead easy, on-your-plate-before-you-know-it recipes. They wouldn't work for me any other way. And I swear, if you don't have any special medical or dietary needs and so can make these recipes a part of your lifestyle, along with following my other tips and doing regular exercise, you will be feeling great before you know it.

RECIPES

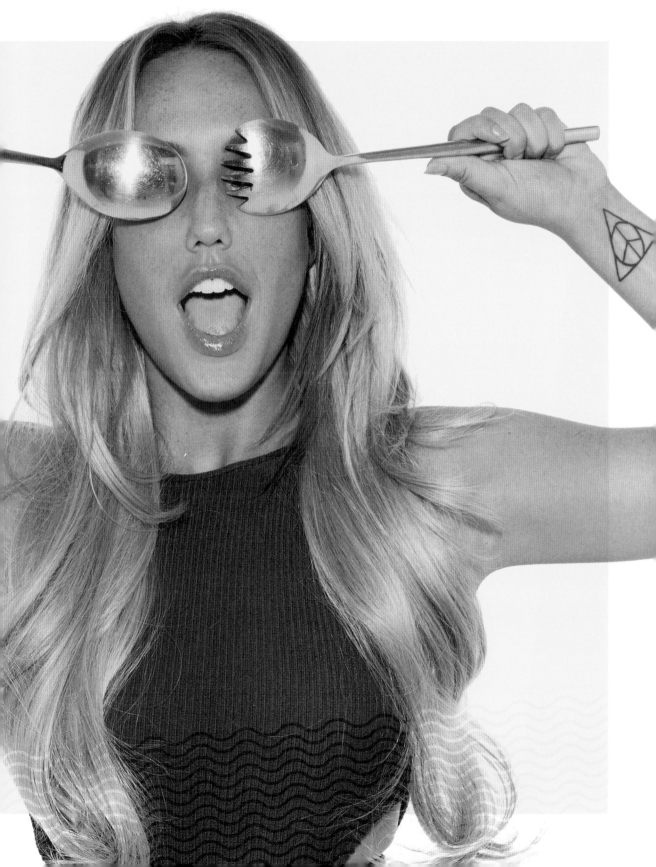

★ THINGS I LIKE TO HAVE IN

In my cupboard

- Black pepper
- Brown rice
- Chilli powder / paprika / cayenne pepper
- Cinnamon powder
- Coconut oil
- Cockles (my favourite snack!)
- Dried mixed herbs / tarragon / oregano
- Eggs
- Fajita seasoning blend
- Garlic
- Ground cumin
- Ground turmeric
- Jalapeños
- Orange juice / apple juice / pomegranate juice
- Olive oil
- Peanut butter (no added sugar)
- Pesto
- Piri piri seasoning blend
- Pitted olives
- Salt

- Soy sauce (or gluten-free tamari)
- Sweet smoked paprika
- Tinned chickpeas / kidney beans / butter beans / mixed beans
- Tinned choppped tomatoes
- Tinned tuna in brine
- Unsweetened almond milk
- Vegetable bouillon powder

In my freezer

- Chopped mango
- Mixed berries / blueberries
- Sliced bananas

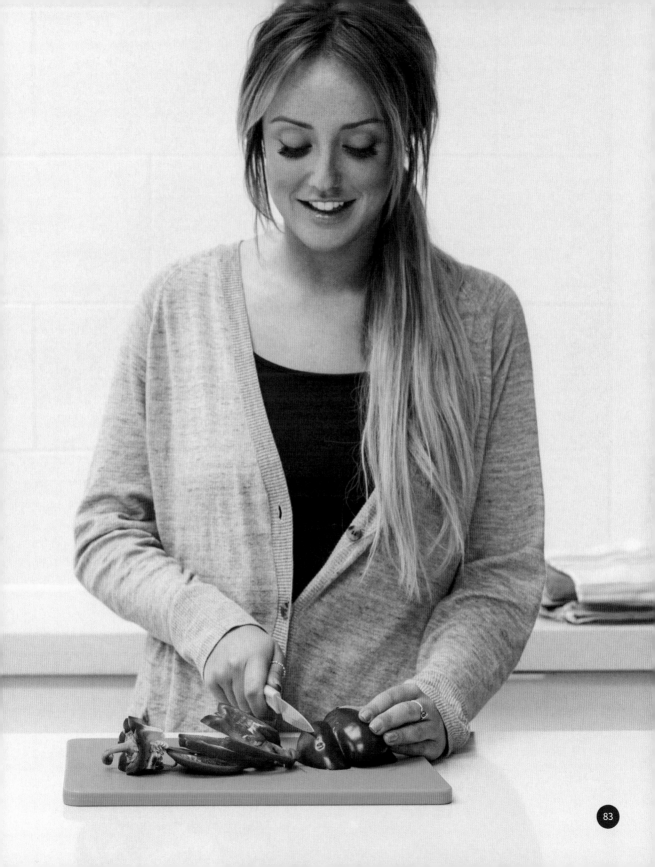

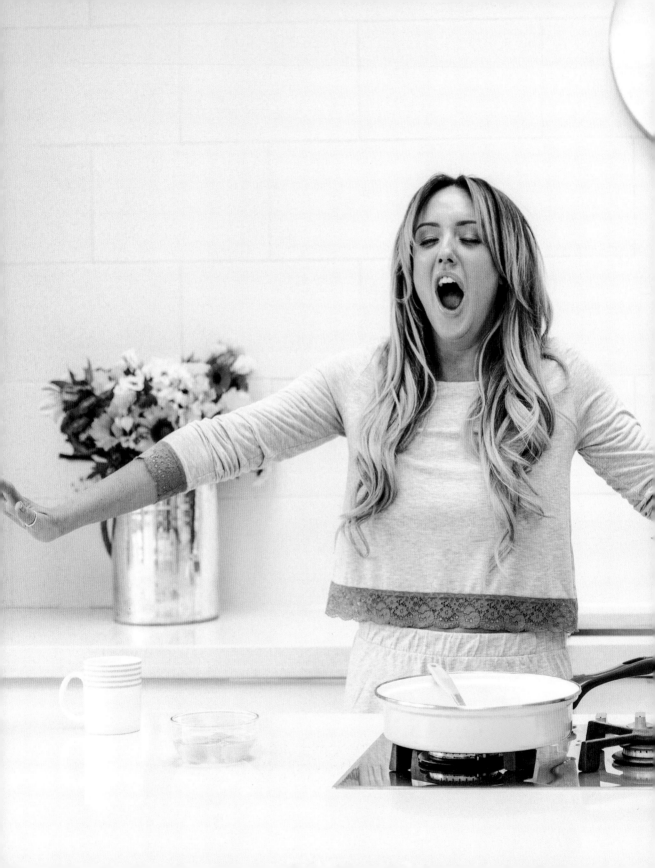

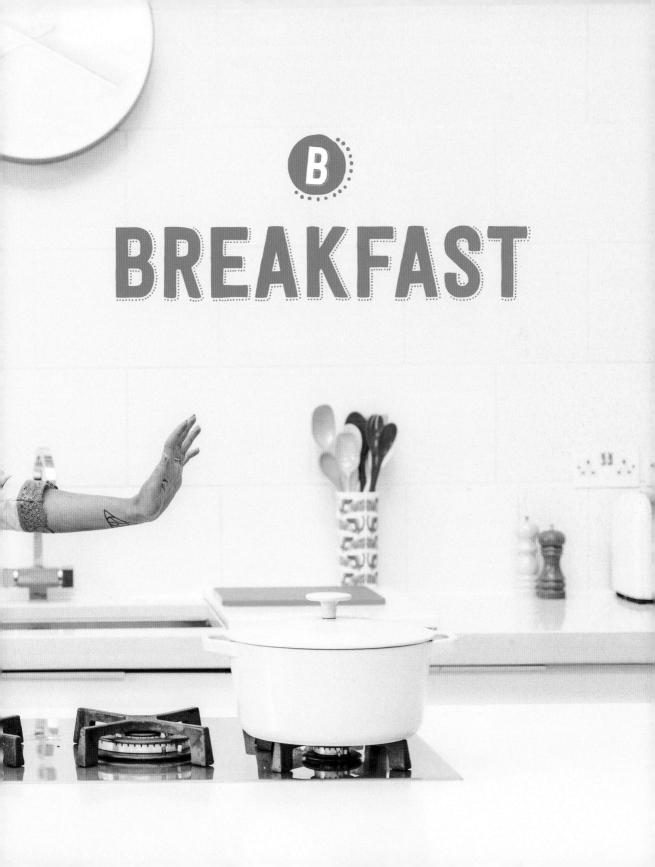

B

BREAKFAST

Classic poached eggs on toast

Serves 1

If you can master a poached egg then you'll always have a simple tasty breakfast you can do easily.

Ingredients
3 medium free-range eggs
1 slice wholemeal, wholegrain or rye bread
salt and black pepper

Fill a saucepan with boiling water from the kettle and place over a medium-low heat so the water is gently bubbling. Put the bread on to toast.

Crack one of the eggs into a cup and use the cup to gently lower the egg into the water. Repeat with the remaining eggs. Cook for 3 minutes, or until cooked to your liking. Remove the eggs from the water with a slotted spoon and hold them over a piece of kitchen paper for a few seconds to drain. Put the toast on a plate and top with the poached eggs. Season with salt and pepper and serve.

TIP: You need very fresh eggs to poach them directly in water. To make poaching eggs easier you can use silicone egg poachers or an egg poaching pan, which keep the eggs intact as they cook.

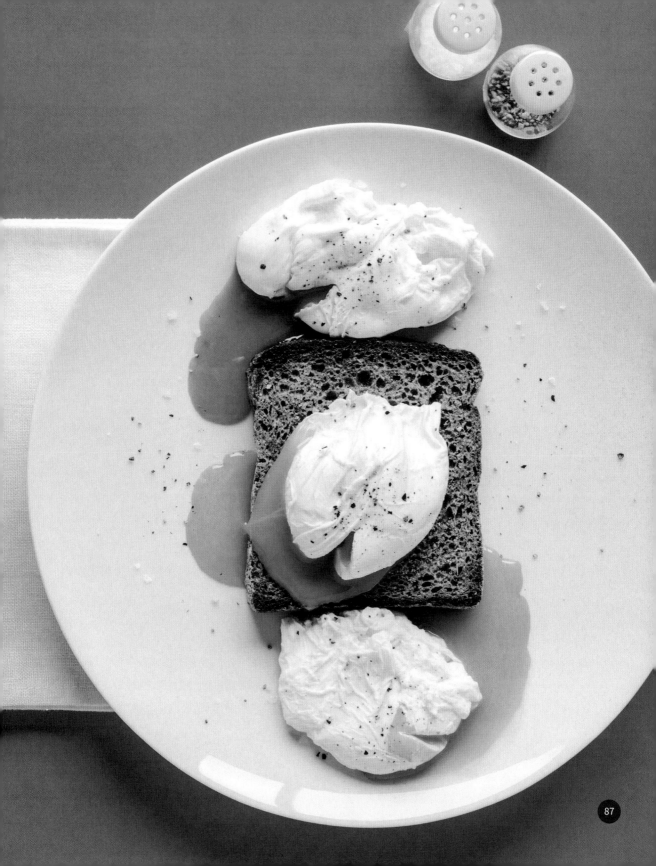

Protein pancakes topped with a fried egg

Serves 1

MAKES 6 PANCAKES

Protein pancakes are my favourite; if I could I'd eat them at any time of the day. At first you might think having them with an egg's not very nice, but trust me, it's amazing.

Ingredients

3 medium free-range eggs
1 banana, peeled and mashed to a gloopy pulp (85g prepared weight)
1 tbsp smooth peanut butter (choose one with no added sugar)
2 tbsp ground almonds
½ tsp baking powder
3 tsp coconut oil, plus 1 tsp for frying the egg

VARIATION

I always have this with a fried egg, but it works just as well with a poached egg. For how to make the perfect poached egg see page 96.

Preheat the oven to 100°C/gas ¼ to keep the pancakes warm while you cook them in batches.

Crack two eggs into a mixing bowl and lightly beat them with a fork. Add the banana, peanut butter, ground almonds and baking powder and beat together with the fork until you have a lumpy batter.

Heat 1 teaspoon of the coconut oil in a large non-stick frying pan over a medium heat. Once it's hot, add large spoonfuls (about 2 tablespoons for each pancake) of the batter to the pan. You should be able to fit two to four pancakes in depending on the size of your pan. Cook until they puff up slightly and small bubbles appear on the surface then flip the pancakes. Cook for a further 1–2 minutes until golden. Put them on a plate in the oven to keep warm. Repeat with the rest of the batter, adding more of the coconut oil as needed.

For the fried egg, add 1 teaspoon of coconut oil to the pan, crack in the remaining egg and fry until cooked to your liking. Slide on top of the pancakes and eat.

Omelette with a choice of fillings

Serves 1

Ingredients

2 tsp coconut oil
½ small red onion, chopped
100g mushrooms, sliced
50g ready-cooked skinless chicken
breast, diced
50g baby spinach
3 medium free-range eggs
salt and black pepper

VARIATION

I chose chicken, mushroom, spinach and red onion here, but you can use anything that you have in the fridge and make your own combinations. Other options would be cherry tomatoes, red onion, peppers, lean ham or ready-cooked turkey.

An omelette is simple and great for using up those bits and pieces in the fridge.

Heat 1 teaspoon of coconut oil in a non-stick frying pan over a medium-high heat. Once it's hot, add the onion, mushrooms and chicken and fry for 3–4 minutes until the onion has softened and the chicken is piping hot. Stir in the spinach and cook for another minute until it wilts. Scrape everything into a bowl.

Add the remaining teaspoon of coconut oil to the pan and lower the heat to medium. Crack the eggs into a mixing bowl and lightly beat them with a fork with some salt and pepper. Pour them into the pan and cook for a minute. When the egg starts to set gently draw it into the middle of the pan using a heatproof spatula, then tip the frying pan so the uncooked egg fills the gaps. Cook for a further 2–3 minutes or until the mixture is almost set.

Spread the filling ingredients on the top then fold the omelette in half, encasing the filling. Cook for a further minute or two then slide onto a plate and serve.

TIP: To make an even quicker dish you can skip frying the filling ingredients. Instead cook the egg as above and scatter the omelette with cold filling ingredients before folding over the omelette.

Fresh fruit layered with yoghurt

Serves 1

This is the easiest breakfast you could possibly make – just use whatever fruit you've got in.

Layer the yoghurt and fruit in a glass or a small bowl.

Serve.

Ingredients

150g 0% fat natural
Greek-style yoghurt
150g prepared fresh fruit
(figs, plums, apples, melon, berries)

VARIATION

Top with 1 tablespoon of chopped,
unblanched (i.e. still in their brown,
papery skins) almonds or pecan nuts.

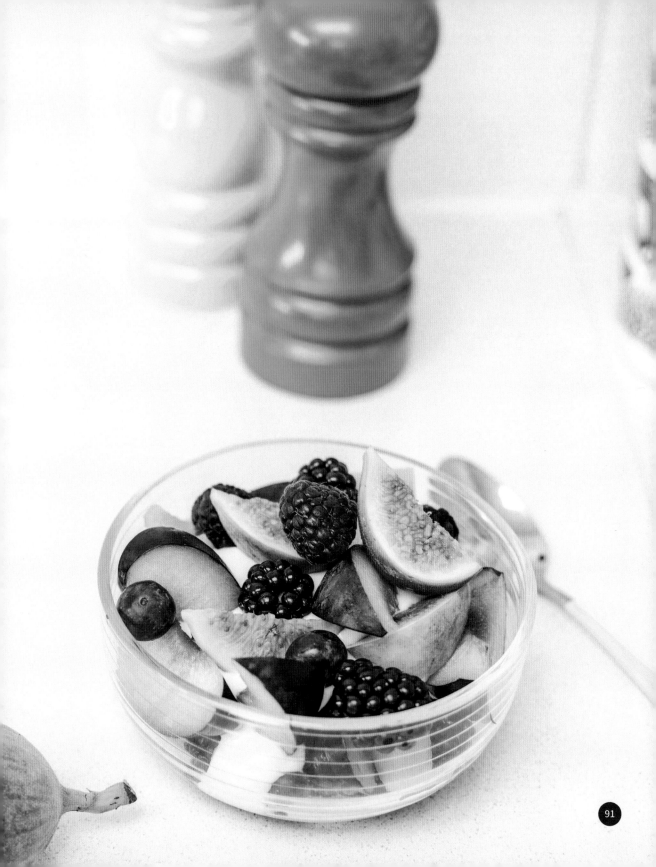

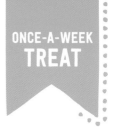

Peanut butter and banana toast

Serves 1

This is really tasty – especially for those of you with a sweet tooth – and dead easy.

Ingredients

1 slice wholemeal, wholegrain or rye bread
1 tbsp crunchy or smooth peanut butter (choose one with no added sugar)
1 banana, peeled and sliced
¼ tsp ground cinnamon (optional)

Toast the bread then spread with the peanut butter.

Top with the banana (mash gently with a fork if you like) and, if you're using it, a sprinkle of cinnamon.

Eat!

Scrambled eggs with spinach, tomatoes and mushrooms

Serves 1

A great low-calorie breakfast that still has enough fuel to get your day kickstarted.

Ingredients
2 tsp coconut oil
50g mushrooms, sliced
50g cherry tomatoes, halved
50g spinach or baby spinach
3 medium free-range eggs
2 tbsp unsweetened almond milk, oat milk or semi-skimmed milk
salt and black pepper

Heat 1 teaspoon of the coconut oil in a non-stick frying pan over a medium heat. Once it's hot, add the mushrooms and fry for 2 minutes then add the tomatoes and fry for another 3–4 minutes or until the mushrooms are lightly browned and the tomatoes have collapsed a bit. Add the spinach and stir for a minute or two until it's wilted. Add a bit of salt and pepper and turn off the heat.

Lightly beat the eggs in a bowl with the milk and a pinch of salt and pepper. In a second frying pan melt the remaining teaspoon of coconut oil over a medium heat. Once it's hot, add the eggs and cook for a minute or two then stir gently once or twice and leave to cook for a minute more, don't stir them so much that they end up in tiny pieces. Repeat this until the eggs are just cooked, but not rubbery.

Serve the scrambled eggs with the vegetables.

TIP: If you have a big frying pan you can cook the eggs next to the vegetables at the same time.

Blueberry protein pancake stack with yoghurt and berries

Serves 1

This is a different take on my favourite protein pancakes, for when I fancy something a bit sweeter.

Ingredients

2 medium free-range eggs
1 banana, peeled and mashed to a gloopy pulp (85g prepared weight)
1 tbsp smooth peanut butter (choose one with no added sugar)
2 tbsp ground almonds
½ tsp baking powder
½ tsp vanilla extract (optional)
2 tsp coconut oil
100g blueberries
2 tbsp 0% fat natural Greek-style yoghurt
a handful of fresh berries (blueberries, raspberries, strawberries)

VARIATION

You could also serve these with sliced banana.

Preheat the oven to 100°C/gas ¼ to keep the pancakes warm while you cook them in batches.

Crack the eggs into a mixing bowl and lightly beat them with a fork. Add the banana, peanut butter, ground almonds and baking powder and, if you're using it, the vanilla extract and beat together with the fork until you have a lumpy batter.

Heat half the coconut oil in a large non-stick frying pan over a medium heat. Once it's hot, add large spoonfuls (about 2 tablespoons for each pancake) of the batter to the pan. You should be able to fit two to four pancakes in depending on the size of your pan. Cook until they puff up slightly and small bubbles appear on the surface then scatter some of the blueberries into the batter and flip the pancakes. Cook for a further 1–2 minutes until golden. Put them on a plate in the oven to keep warm while you cook the rest. Repeat with the rest of the batter, adding more coconut oil as you need it.

Stack the pancakes up, top with yoghurt and your choice of berries, then eat.

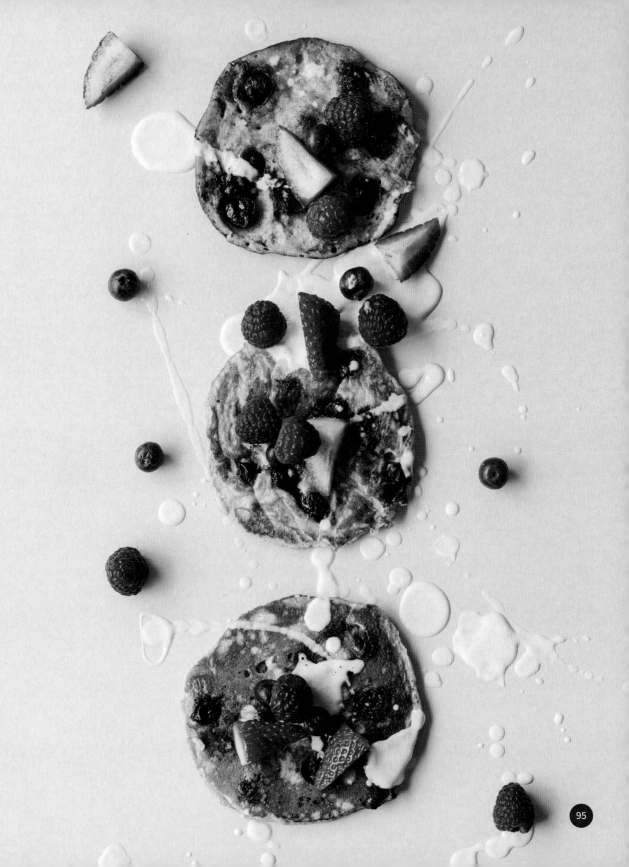

Brekkie hash

Serves 1

This one is a great fuel booster for when you're exercising, and is packed full with loads of different flavours.

Ingredients
1–2 tsp coconut oil
75g cherry tomatoes, halved
100g mushrooms, sliced
50g lean ham, all fat trimmed off and finely chopped
50g baby spinach
3 medium free-range eggs
salt and black pepper

Heat 1 teaspoon of the coconut oil in a non-stick frying pan over a medium heat. Once it's hot, add the tomatoes and mushrooms and fry for 3–4 minutes until the mushrooms are just golden. Stir in the ham and fry for a minute, then add the spinach and cook for a further minute until it wilts.

Make three small gaps in the pan. If the pan looks dry then add a little of the remaining coconut oil into each gap. Crack one of the eggs into a cup and pour into one of the gaps. Repeat with the remaining eggs. Season each egg with a pinch of salt and pepper.

Cover the pan with a lid and cook for 3–4 minutes, or until the eggs are cooked to your liking. Remove from pan with a fish slice and slide onto a plate, don't worry if it breaks up as you do this.

TIP: If you don't have a big enough lid for your frying pan you can cover it with a baking tray or a second frying pan, or pop the pan under a medium preheated grill for a minute or two.

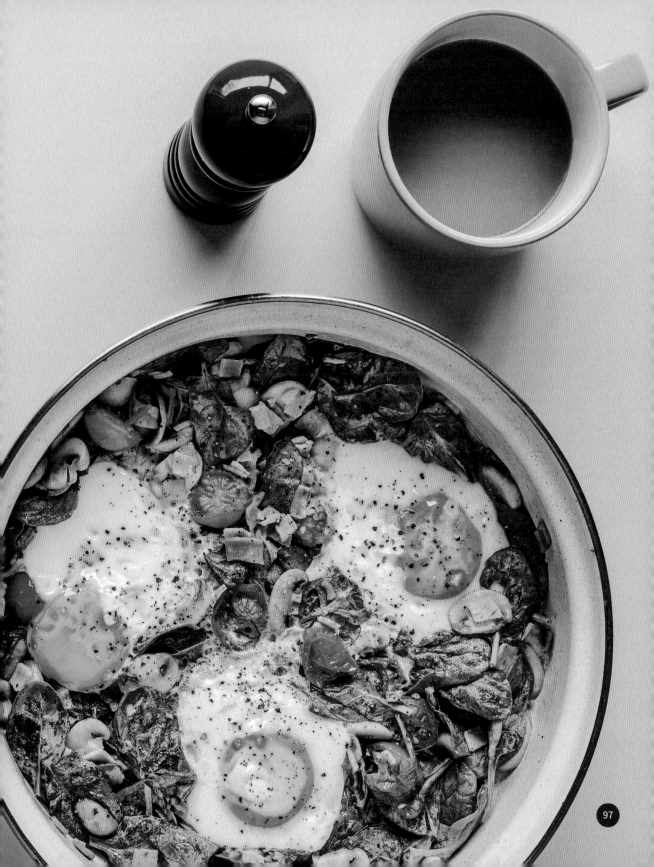

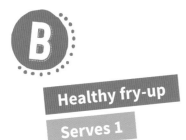

Healthy fry-up

Serves 1

A fry-up is one of my favourites – so it's good to know I can still have one even when I'm trying to lose weight.

Ingredients

3 turkey rashers
2 medium tomatoes, halved
2 tsp coconut oil
100g mushrooms, sliced
2 medium free-range eggs
1 tbsp unsweetened almond milk, oat milk or semi-skimmed milk
salt and black pepper

Preheat the grill to medium-high. Place the turkey rashers and the tomatoes, cut-side-up, on a baking tray or grill pan. Season the tomatoes with salt and pepper. Place the pan under the grill. After 2 minutes turn the turkey rashers over and grill for a further 2 minutes before removing from the grill pan. Grill the tomatoes for a further 3–4 minutes or until softened. Set aside.

Meanwhile, heat 1 teaspoon of the coconut oil in a non-stick frying pan over a medium heat. Once it's hot, add the mushrooms with a pinch of salt and pepper and fry for 5–6 minutes until softened and browned at the edges. Tip onto a plate and keep warm underneath the grill.

Wipe round the frying pan with a piece of kitchen towel, add the remaining teaspoon of coconut oil and lower the heat to medium-low. Crack the eggs into a bowl, add the milk and some salt and pepper and whisk lightly with a fork. Pour the eggs into the frying pan, cook for a minute then stir gently. Leave to cook for a minute or two longer, then stir again gently until they are in soft folds.

When the eggs are cooked serve them on the plate next to the mushrooms. Add the turkey rashers and tomatoes.

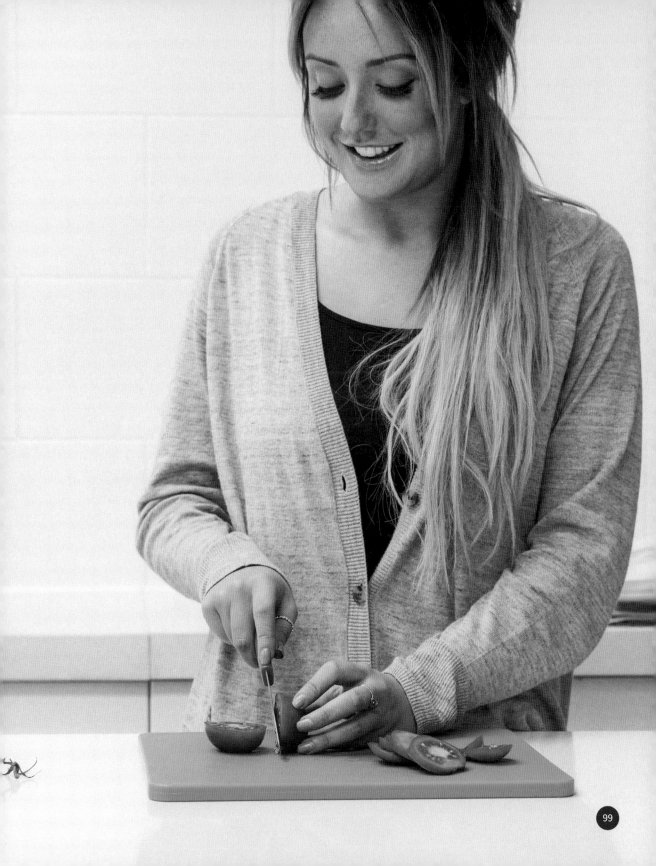

Banana and cinnamon omelette

Serves 1

Ingredients

1 tsp coconut oil
3 medium free-range eggs
salt
1 tsp ground cinnamon
1 banana, peeled and sliced

This is another one that sounds a bit odd and crazy, but it tastes amazing and is something a little bit different.

Heat the coconut oil in a non-stick frying pan over a medium heat. Crack the eggs into a mixing bowl and lightly beat them with a fork with a small pinch of salt and half the cinnamon. Pour them into the pan and cook for a minute. When the egg starts to set gently draw it from the edges into the middle of the pan using a heatproof spatula, then tip the frying pan so the uncooked egg fills the gaps. Cook for a further 2–3 minutes or until the mixture is almost set.

Scatter the banana on top then fold the omelette in half, encasing the banana. Cook for a further minute or two then slide onto a plate. Sprinkle with the remaining cinnamon and serve.

Porridge with honey

Serves 1

Porridge is best for a day when you know you're going to be exercising as it's full of good carbs.

Ingredients
50g porridge oats
300ml unsweetened almond milk,
oat milk or semi-skimmed milk
½ tsp clear, runny honey

VARIATION

You could top the porridge with a sliced banana and a sprinkle of ground cinnamon or ½ teaspoon of desiccated or shaved coconut. Try stirring in a coarsely grated apple and topping with 1 teaspoon of chopped walnuts or pecan nuts. Or simply add a handful of fresh berries.

Mix the oats with the milk in a saucepan over a medium heat. Once it begins to bubble, reduce the heat slightly and simmer for 2–3 minutes, or until thick and creamy. If it's too thin then cook for a little longer. If it's too thick then add a splash of boiling water.

Serve drizzled with the honey.

Veggie fritters with poached eggs

Serves 1

I love this recipe because it's a bit different and exciting, for times when you're getting bored of the same old options.

Ingredients

3 medium free-range eggs
1 small carrot, coarsely grated
1 small courgette, coarsely grated
1 tbsp plain flour
2 tsp coconut oil
salt and black pepper

Fill a saucepan with boiling water from the kettle and place over a medium-low heat so the water is gently bubbling.

For the fritters, crack one egg into a mixing bowl and lightly beat with a fork. Add the carrot, courgette and flour, season with salt and pepper, and mix together.

Heat the coconut oil in a non-stick frying pan over a medium heat. Once it's hot, add large spoonfuls of the vegetable mixture to the pan, making two or three fritters (you might need to cook them in batches if your pan is small). Fry for 3–4 minutes, or until golden underneath, then flip and cook for another 2–3 minutes until golden.

While the fritters are cooking you can poach your other two eggs. Crack one egg into a cup then gently lower the egg into the water. Repeat with the remaining egg. Cook for 3 minutes then remove the eggs with a slotted spoon and drain over a piece of kitchen paper.

SEE TIP
ON PAGE
96

Put the fritters on a plate and top with the poached eggs. Serve.

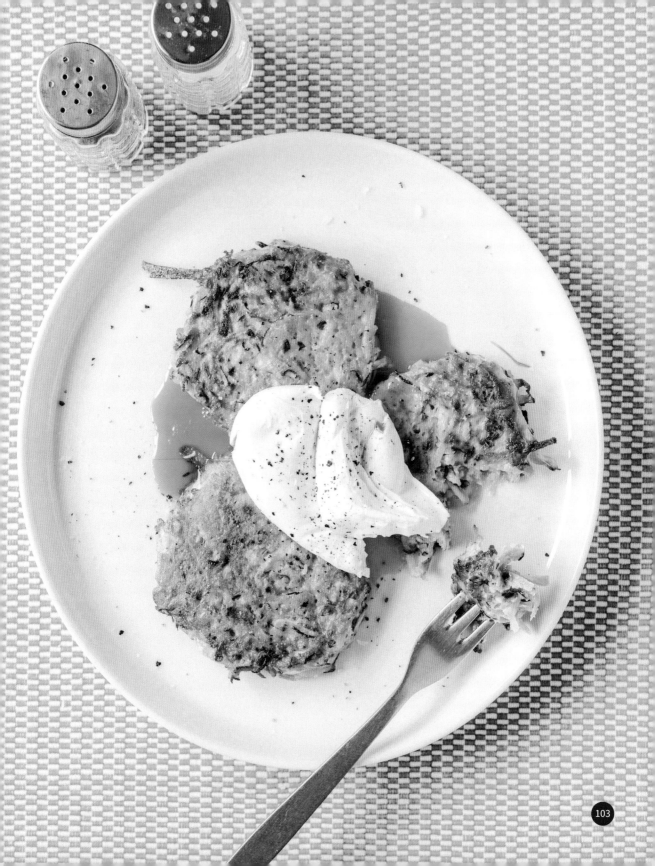

Chorizo mini muffins

Serves 3–4

The great thing about these is that you can freeze them for up to a month so when I make twelve I just eat three or four and freeze the rest for another day when I'm in a rush.

Ingredients

1 tsp coconut oil
50g cooking chorizo or cured chorizo, finely chopped
1 medium red onion, thinly sliced
6 medium free-range eggs
2 tbsp 0% fat natural Greek-style yoghurt
80g soft or crumbly goats' cheese
1 tsp paprika or chilli powder
black pepper

VARIATION

For a veggie option, leave out the chorizo and add half a finely diced red pepper with the onion.

Pre-heat the oven to 180°C/gas 4. Put the coconut oil in one of the wells of a 12-hole non-stick muffin tin. Put it in the oven for a minute until the coconut oil has melted then use a pastry brush or a piece of kitchen paper to grease the inside of all the wells with the oil.

Place roughly equal amounts of chorizo in each well then repeat with the onion. Cook in the oven for 6–8 minutes until sizzling.

Meanwhile crack the eggs into a bowl. Add the yoghurt, season with pepper and beat with a fork.

Remove the tin from the oven and pour the egg mixture into each hole. Top each with some of the goats' cheese and a sprinkle of paprika then return to the oven and bake for 15 minutes. Serve hot or cold.

TIP: You can buy ready-diced chorizo in most supermarkets to save time.

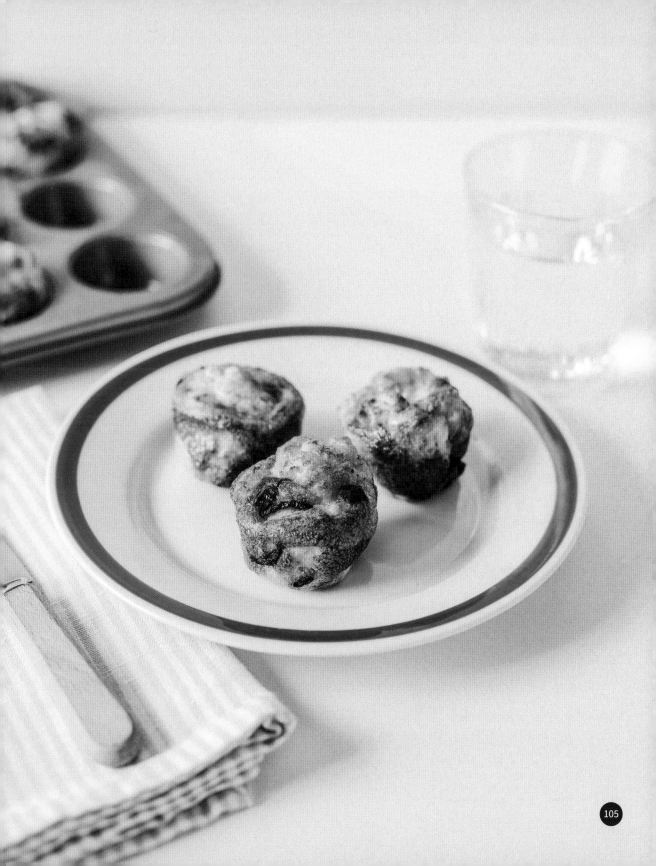

Poached eggs with ham and wilted spinach

Serves 1

Ingredients
100g baby spinach
2 slices (75–100g) lean ham,
all fat trimmed off
3 medium free-range eggs
black pepper

I eat a lot of spinach – for breakfast, lunch and dinner!

Rinse the spinach and put it into a saucepan, with the water still clinging to it, and cover with a lid. Cook over a medium heat for 1 minute or until just wilted. Transfer to a plate. Rinse the pan then fill it with boiling water from the kettle and return to a medium-low heat so the water is gently bubbling.

Crack one of the eggs into a cup and gently lower the egg into the water. Repeat with the remaining eggs. Cook for 3 minutes, or until cooked to your liking. Remove the eggs from the water with a slotted spoon and hold them over a piece of kitchen paper for a few seconds to drain.

Place the slices of ham on a plate and pile the spinach on top. Finish with the poached eggs and season with black pepper.

SEE TIP ON PAGE 96

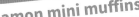
Banana, oat and cinnamon mini muffins

Serves 3–4

Ingredients
1½ tsp coconut oil
1½ bananas, peeled and mashed
(130g prepared weight)
1 large apple, peeled, cored and
coarsely grated
3 medium free-range eggs
40g porridge oats
1½ tsp ground cinnamon

VARIATION

If you want to add more banana then peel and chop a second banana and scatter on top of the mixture once it's in the muffin tin and bake as per instructions.

These are fun and it feels like you're eating cake even though you're not – so it's a win-win situation.

Pre-heat the oven to 200°C/gas 6. Put the coconut oil in one of the wells of a 12-hole non-stick muffin tin. Put it in the oven for a minute until the coconut oil has melted then use a pastry brush or a piece of kitchen paper to grease the inside of all the wells with the oil.

In a bowl mix together all the remaining ingredients. Divide them between the greased wells and bake for 12 minutes or until golden and just firm to the touch. Eat them warm or cold.

TIP: You can bake one large 'muffin' (which will look more like a thin cake) in pretty much any non-stick tin or even a baking dish (aim for roughly an 18-cm round tin or a 15-cm square tin). You'll need to bake it for 15 minutes.

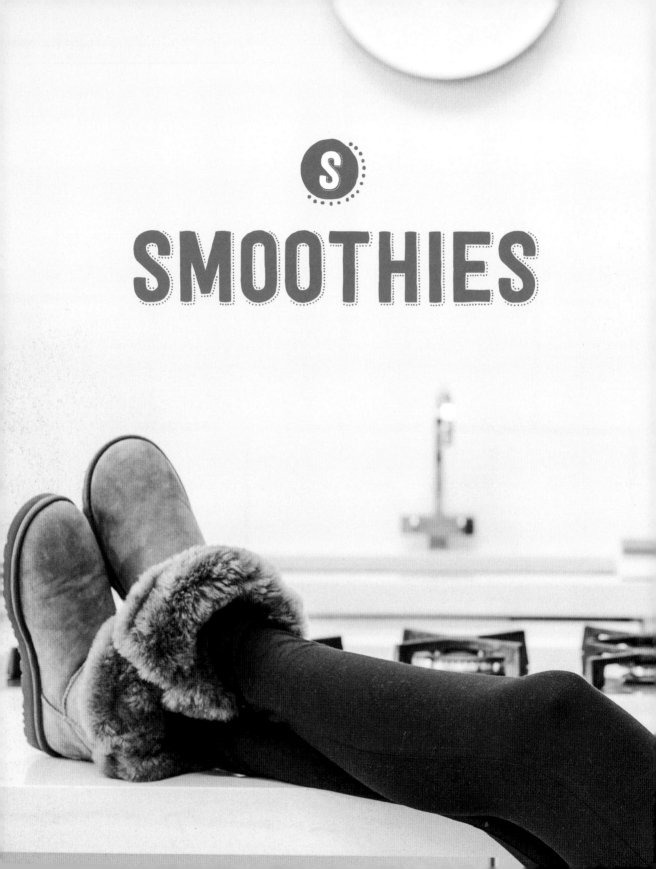

SMOOTHIES

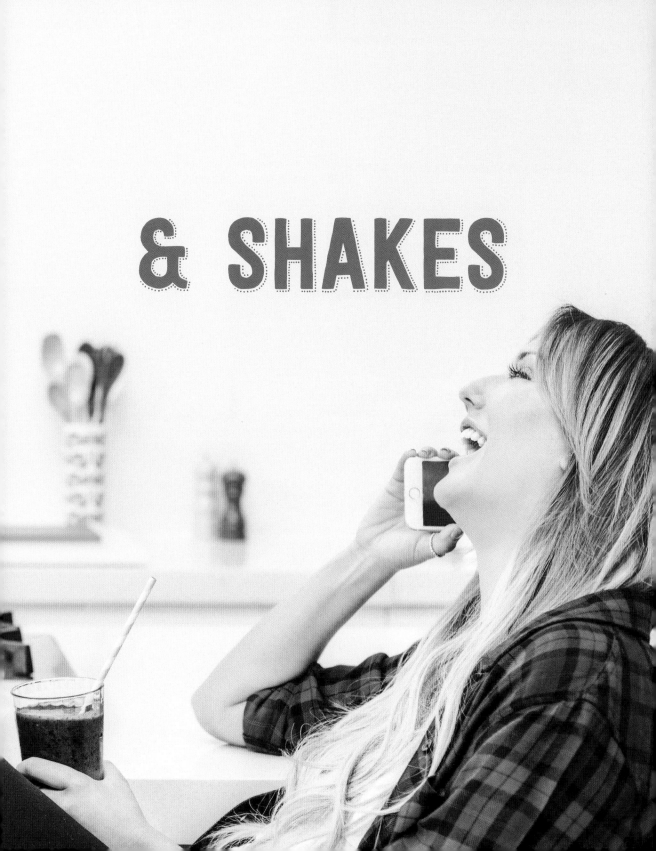

Berry smoothie

Serves 1

Ingredients

150g frozen mixed berries
(strawberries, raspberries,
blueberries)
150ml unsweetened 100%
pomegranate juice or orange juice
2 tsp almond butter (optional)

I love smoothies for a quick fill-up when I'm on the go or in a rush, but you should never have more than one in a day, and I avoid eating any other sweet things that day if I've had one.

Put the berries, 150ml of the juice and the almond butter, if you have it, into a blender and blitz until thick and smooth, add a splash of water if needed.

Pour into a glass and drink straight away.

TIP: You can buy bags of frozen berries to keep in your freezer ready to make a quick smoothie.

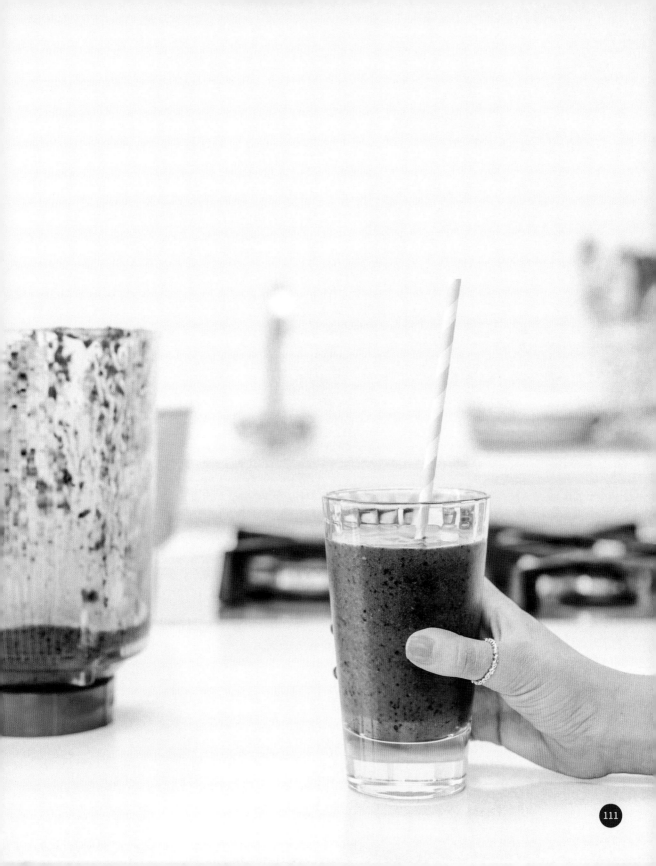

Banana and oat shake

Serves 1

This is one my trainer recommends as the banana and oats release energy slowly, so great for a training day.

Ingredients
150–175ml unsweetened almond milk, oat milk or semi-skimmed milk
1 banana, peeled, chopped and frozen
50g 0% fat natural Greek-style yoghurt
2 oatcakes (20g), crumbled or 20g porridge oats
1 tbsp smooth or crunchy peanut butter (choose one with no added sugar)

Tip everything into a blender with 150ml of the milk and blitz to a smooth, thick consistency. Add more milk if needed.

Pour into a glass and drink straight away.

SEE TIP OPPOSITE

Spinach, blueberry and pomegranate smoothie

Serves 1

I love blueberries and they add a fruity burst to this smoothy. You're sure to enjoy it.

Ingredients
35g baby spinach
50g frozen blueberries
½ banana, peeled, chopped and frozen
150ml unsweetened 100% pomegranate juice

Tip everything into a blender with 175ml of the pomegranate juice and blitz to a smooth, thick consistency. Add more juice if needed. Add a splash of water if needed.

Pour into a glass and drink straight away.

TIP: You can buy frozen blueberries in the supermarket, or you can add a handful of ice cubes to the blender.

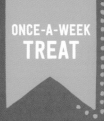

Chocolate avocado thick shake

Serves 1

Ingredients
½ ripe avocado
½ banana, peeled, chopped and frozen
1 tbsp unsweetened cocoa powder
½ tsp vanilla extract (optional)
½ small square dark chocolate (5g), chopped (optional)
100–150ml unsweetened almond milk, oat milk or semi-skimmed milk

VARIATION

For a bit of a blow-out, you can add 1 tablespoon of peanut butter (choose one with no added sugar) to give it extra protein – but this makes it more of a treat, or a filling breakfast.

In this shake I allow myself a little bit of my favourite dark chocolate.

Cut the avocado in half, remove the stone and scoop out the flesh into a blender. Add all the other ingredients and 100ml of the milk. Blitz to a smooth, thick consistency, adding a little more milk if necessary.

Pour into a glass and drink straight away while thick and ice cold.

TIP: Freeze the chopped banana for at least a few hours beforehand for an extra thick, icy smoothie. I keep a stash of frozen, chopped banana in my freezer for smoothies, shakes and my Banana and dark chocolate ice cream (see page 202). If you don't have any frozen then add a handful of ice cubes to the blender.

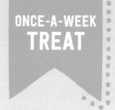

Frozen mango and banana smoothie

Serves 1

The banana makes this a good pick-me-up if you're feeling low on energy.

Ingredients

75g mango, peeled, chopped and frozen
¾ banana, peeled, chopped and frozen
150ml cloudy apple juice or orange juice
½ tbsp lime juice, or juice of ½ lime (optional)

Tip the mango and banana into a blender with 150ml of the juice and blitz to a smooth, thick consistency. Add the lime juice, if using, and a splash of water if needed.

Pour into a glass and drink straight away.

TIP: Keep a stash of chopped banana and chopped mango in your freezer for this smoothie. You can buy frozen mango in supermarkets.

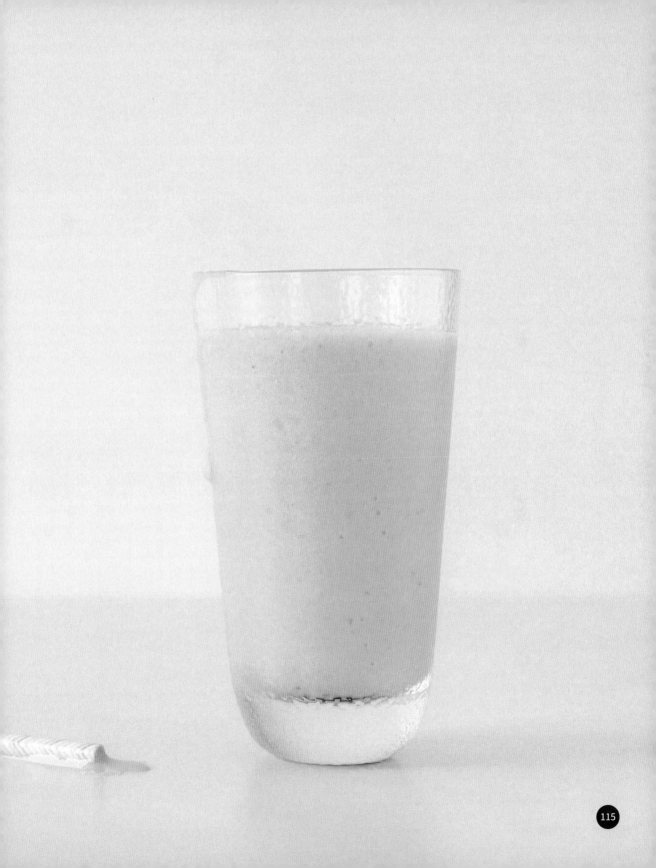

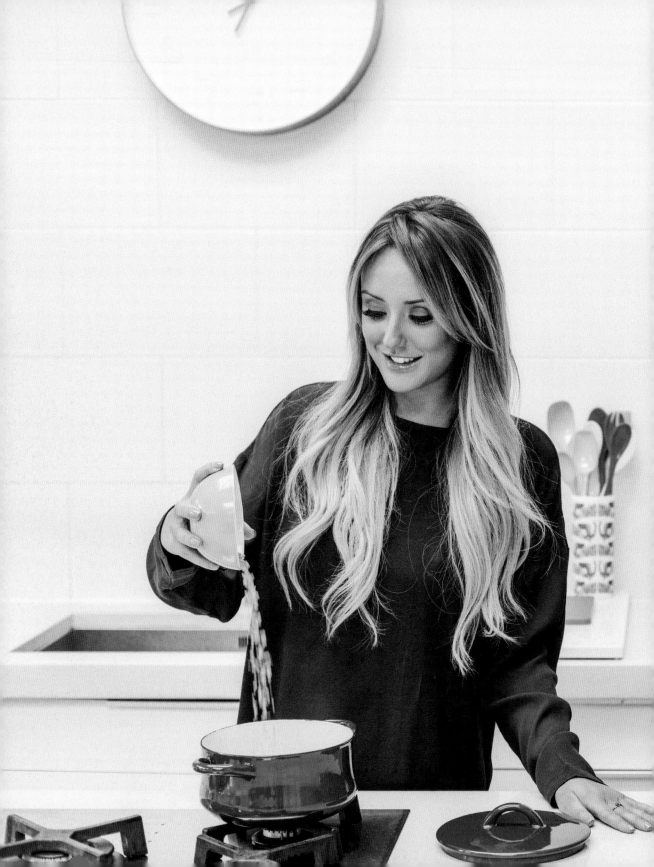

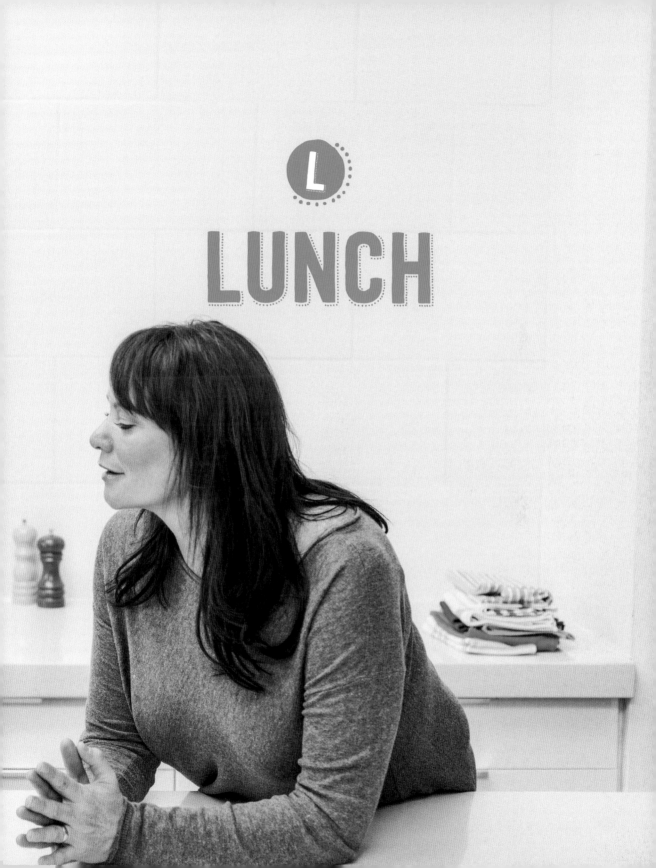

LUNCH

Letitia's soup done the Charlotte way

Serves 2

Me mam's been making this for years – I love it.

Ingredients
50g red lentils, rinsed
50g pearl barley, rinsed
1 large leek, rinsed and cut into 2-cm chunks (110g prepared weight)
400g root vegetables (carrots, sweet potatoes, parsnips, swede), peeled and diced
100g lean back bacon or gammon steak, all fat trimmed off and diced
1 tsp vegetable bouillon powder
750ml boiling water
black pepper

Put all the ingredients into a saucepan or flameproof casserole. Bring to a boil then lower the heat, cover and simmer over a low heat for one hour, stirring occasionally and adding more boiling water if it looks dry.

Season with black pepper and serve in warmed bowls.

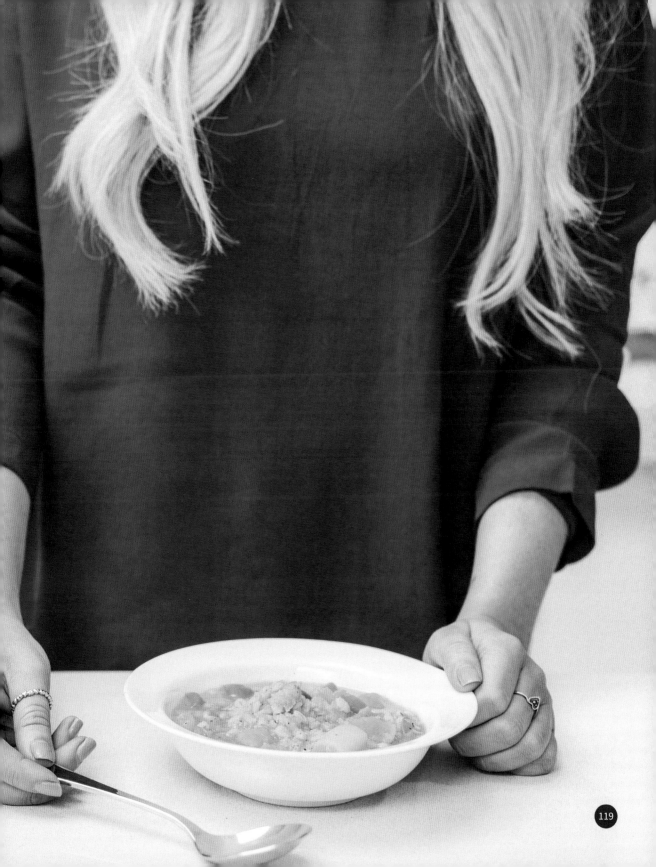

Salmon and pesto salad

Serves 1

This is a really quick one and is perfect for lunch on the go.

Ingredients
50g salad leaves
50g cherry tomatoes, quartered
50g mushrooms, thinly sliced
1 heaped tsp ready-made pesto
80–100g ready-cooked salmon or trout fillet, skin removed
black pepper

In a bowl, gently mix together the salad leaves, tomatoes, mushrooms and pesto. Leave for a few minutes to allow the flavours to combine. Flake the salmon into large pieces and scatter on top of the salad. Grind over some black pepper and serve.

TIP: You can make this the night before and leave in the fridge to take as a packed lunch the following day.

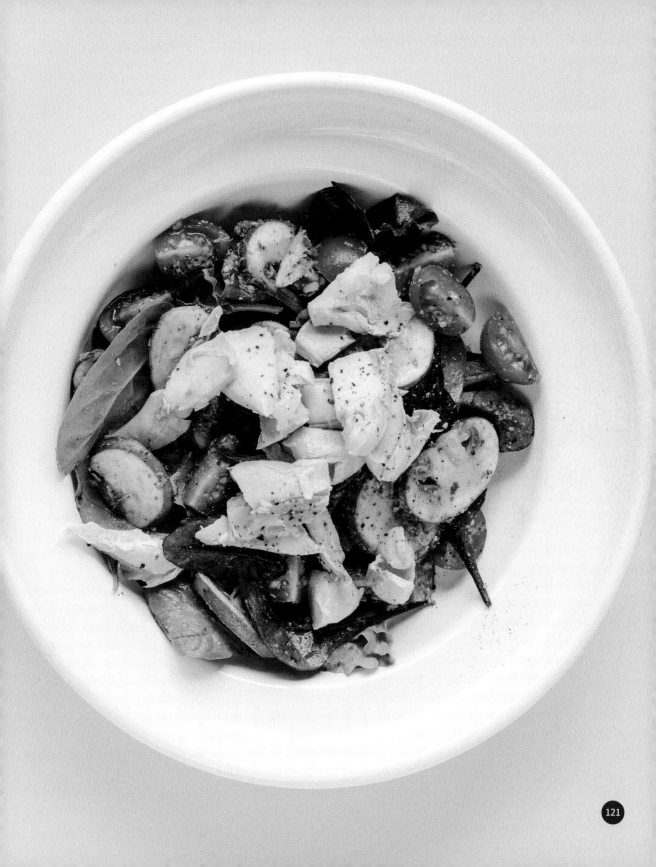

Tuna mayo and olive salad

Serves 1

As you know, I *love* olives and they contrast really well with the tuna in this salad.

Ingredients

35g salad leaves or crisp lettuce, torn
100g tin tuna in brine, drained
(60–75g drained weight)
2–3 tsp light mayonnaise
½ small red onion, finely chopped
½ tsp dried chilli flakes
black pepper
1 tbsp lemon juice or juice of ½
lemon (optional)
25g pitted black olives, halved or
left whole

VARIATION

Also good with a chopped hard-boiled egg on top if you need extra protein.

Put the salad leaves on a plate. In a bowl, mix together the tuna, mayonnaise, onion, chilli and black pepper. Add the lemon juice too, if using. Spoon on top of the salad leaves and scatter with the black olives. Serve.

Mixed bean, tuna, red onion and chilli salad

Serves 1–2

Depending on how much chilli you add, this can really get your nose running!

Ingredients
400g tin mixed beans,
drained and rinsed
200g tin tuna in brine, drained
(150g drained weight)
1 small red onion, finely chopped
1 tbsp lime juice, or juice of 1 lime
½–1 tsp mild chilli powder
black pepper

Mix everything together in a large bowl, adding the chilli powder to your taste, and plenty of black pepper. Serve or cover and keep in the fridge overnight.

Four seasons salad

Serves 1

All the flavours of your favourite pizza topping – but as a healthy salad instead.

Ingredients
55g lean ham, all fat trimmed
off and chopped
75g button or chestnut mushrooms,
thinly sliced
½ red pepper, seeds removed, diced
1 tbsp pitted black olives, sliced
2 tsp ready-made pesto
50g salad leaves

Mix the ham, mushrooms, pepper and olives with the pesto and leave to mingle for 5 minutes. Put the salad leaves in a bowl and top with the pesto mixture to serve.

Red pepper and tomato soup

Serves 2

Soups are great light bites and this is one you can keep in the fridge or freezer.

Ingredients

1 small red onion, peeled and cut into quarters
350g medium tomatoes, cut into quarters
2 red peppers, seeds removed, halved
2 cloves garlic
black pepper
2 tsp olive oil
1 tsp smoked paprika (optional)
1 tsp vegetable bouillon powder
350ml boiling water
2 tbsp 0% fat natural Greek-style yoghurt (optional)

Preheat the oven to 200°C/gas 6.

Tip the onion, tomatoes, peppers and garlic into a non-stick roasting tin with some black pepper and the olive oil and toss everything together. Cook in the oven for 20 minutes or until the vegetables are soft.

Squeeze the garlic from its papery skin. Scrape all of the vegetables, including the garlic, into a blender. Add the paprika, if using, the bouillon powder and the boiling water and blitz until smooth. Add more boiling water if needed to get the consistency you like.

Reheat as needed and serve with an optional spoonful of yoghurt and some pepper on top. Eat with some toasted rye bread.

TIP: If you prefer you can scrape the roasted vegetables into a saucepan, add the bouillon powder and boiling water and blend using a stick blender.

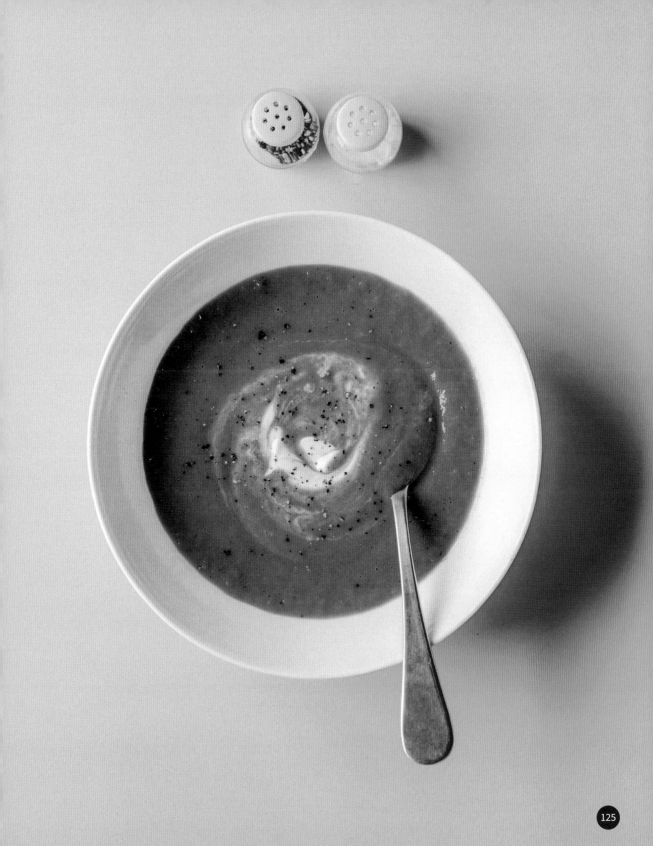

Asian chicken salad with green beans and red onion

Serves 1

It's really easy to double this one up, so it's one to make if you've got a friend over for lunch.

Ingredients
100g mangetout, green beans or sugar snaps
50–75g ready-cooked skinless chicken breast, thinly sliced or shredded
35g baby spinach
½ small red onion, thinly sliced
½ fresh red chilli, thinly sliced
1 tbsp lime juice, or juice of 1 lime
1 heaped tsp crunchy peanut butter (choose one with no added sugar)
1 tsp dark soy sauce or tamari

Cook the mangetout, green beans or sugar snaps in a pan of boiling water over a high heat for 2–3 minutes, or until just cooked but still crunchy. Drain well and rinse under cold water until cool.

Toss together with the chicken, spinach, red onion and chilli.

For the dressing, whisk the lime juice, peanut butter and soy sauce together with a fork, adding 1 teaspoon of boiling water if it's too thick, then spoon over the salad.

Serve.

TIP: To speed things up, the sugar snaps and mangetout can be left raw, but if you are using green beans these do need cooking first.

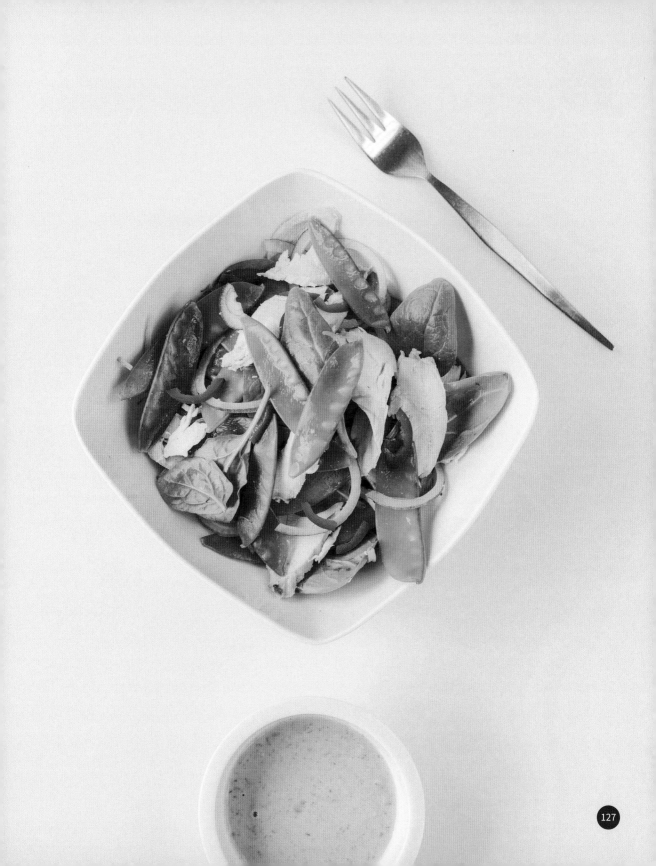

Healthy egg mayo salad

Serves 1

This one I came across totally by accident when I mushed up some eggs with my hummus salad. It was so tasty I had to include it in the book.

Ingredients

2 medium free-range eggs
2 tbsp hummus
black pepper
½ small red onion, finely chopped (optional)
1 little gem lettuce, roughly torn
a pinch of chilli powder or cayenne pepper (optional)

Put a saucepan of water on to boil. Once boiling turn the heat to medium so the water is gently bubbling. Use a spoon to carefully lower in the eggs and boil for 7–8 minutes. Remove from the heat, pour off the water then fill the saucepan with cold water and leave the eggs to cool for a few minutes.

Peel the eggs and put in a bowl. Mash roughly with a fork then stir in the hummus, black pepper and the onion, if using. Put the lettuce on a plate and top with the egg mixture. Sprinkle with a little chilli powder or cayenne pepper, or some more black pepper. Serve with a slice of rye bread.

TIP: You can use any crunchy lettuce for this recipe – you need a small bowlful.

Stuffed roast peppers

Serves 1

If I want a really nice lunch I'll do a stuffed roast pepper with whatever I've got in, so feel free to vary the recipe with whatever is in your fridge.

Ingredients

1 large red pepper, seeds removed, halved
2 tsp coconut oil
1 small onion, chopped
75g mushrooms, chopped
125g lean minced beef (less than 5% fat if you can get it)
½ tsp chilli powder
1 tsp ground cumin
400g tin chopped tomatoes
25g mozzarella or soft or crumbly goats' cheese
salt and black pepper

Preheat the oven to 200°C/gas 6.

Put the red pepper halves in a baking dish, cut side up, and roast in the oven for 10 minutes.

While the pepper halves are cooking, heat the coconut oil in a non-stick frying pan over a medium heat. Once it's hot, add the onion and mushrooms and fry for 5 minutes. Stir in the mince, increase the heat to medium-high, and cook for 2–3 minutes until browned slightly. Stir in the spices followed by the tomatoes and some salt and pepper. Bubble over a medium-high heat, stirring often, for 10 minutes.

Spoon the mince mixture into the pepper halves, top with the cheese and bake in the oven for 10 minutes until the cheese is melted and bubbling. Eat straight away.

Oriental spicy chicken broth

Serves 1

For when I fancy a Chinese takeaway but know I shouldn't have one!

Ingredients

400ml boiling water
½ tsp vegetable bouillon powder
30g spring greens, savoy cabbage or kale, shredded
1 clove garlic, peeled and thinly sliced
2-cm piece root ginger, peeled and thinly sliced
50g ready-cooked skinless chicken breast, diced or shredded
½ fresh red chilli, thinly sliced, or ½ tsp dried chilli flakes
½ tsp dark soy sauce or tamari
black pepper

Put the boiling water into a saucepan and stir in the bouillon powder. Add the greens, garlic and ginger. Cover and bubble over a medium-high heat for 2 minutes.

Stir in the chicken and chilli, cover and bubble for 4 minutes or until the chicken is piping hot. Stir in the soy sauce or tamari, season with black pepper and serve.

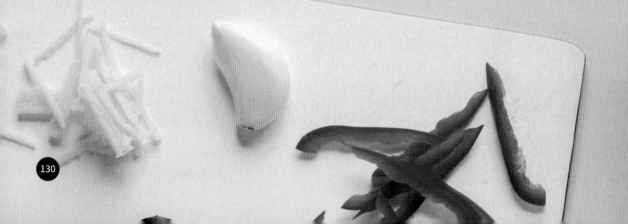

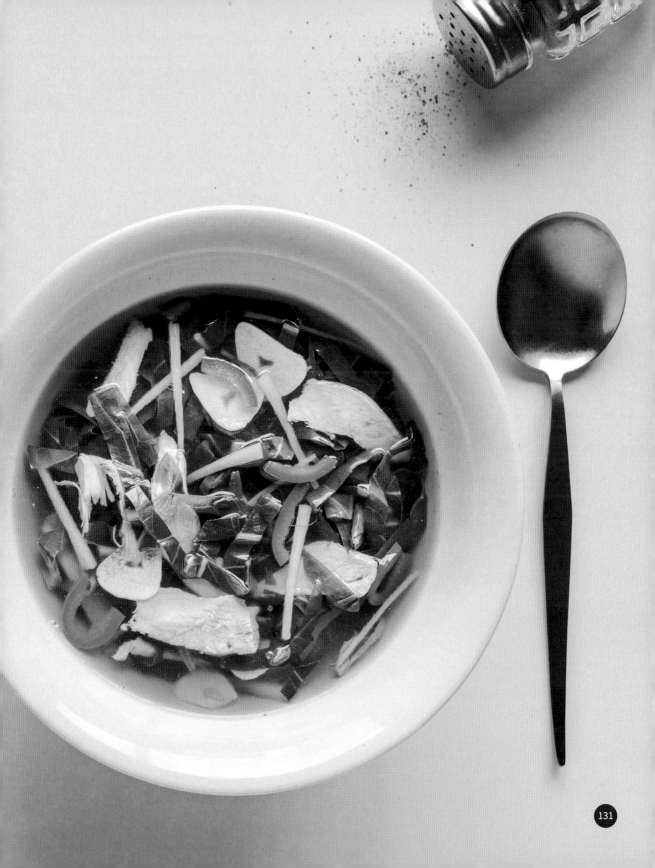

Chicken salad with a bit of everything

Serves 1

This is another really easy salad that you can make if you've not got much time.

Ingredients

35g salad leaves
50–75g ready-cooked skinless chicken breast, chopped or shredded
50g mushrooms, sliced
50g cherry tomatoes, halved
1 small red pepper, seeds removed, diced
½ small red onion, finely chopped
3 tbsp hummus

Put the salad leaves in the bottom of a bowl.

In a second bowl, mix all the remaining ingredients together, then place on top of the salad leaves to serve.

VARIATION

You can also add olives, baby spinach, cucumber or celery to this salad.

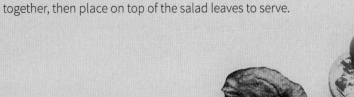

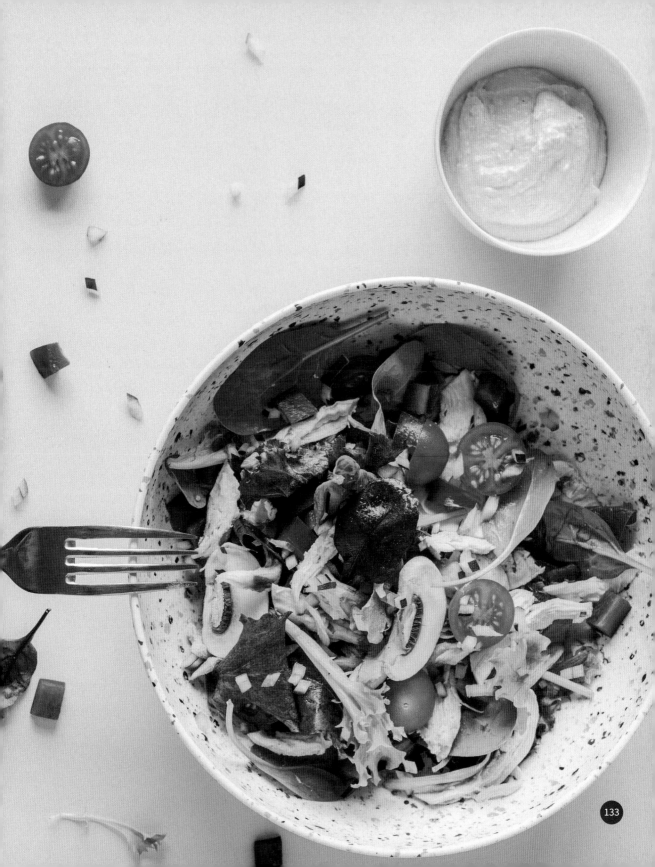

Prawn and avocado salad with Dijon dressing

Serves 1

I love all seafood, and prawns taste great with avocado tossed in a salad.

Ingredients

1 tbsp hummus
1 tsp Dijon mustard
1 tsp lemon juice (optional)
1–2 tsp boiling water
30g baby spinach and/or salad leaves
1 ripe avocado
100g ready-cooked, peeled king prawns or small prawns
black pepper

For the dressing, stir together the hummus and Dijon mustard, and the lemon juice, if using, with the boiling water to get a smooth, creamy dressing.

Put the salad leaves on a plate. Cut the avocado in half, remove the stone and peel away the skin, or scoop out the flesh using a spoon. Slice the flesh.

Put the sliced avocado on top of the leaves with a pile of prawns alongside. Grind over some black pepper then drizzle over the dressing and eat.

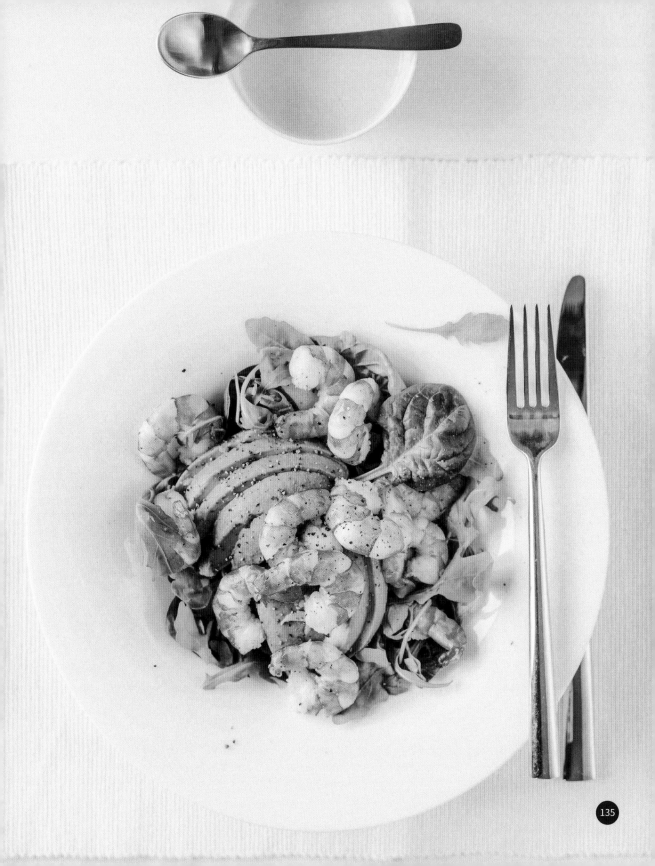

Curried sweet potato soup

Serves 2

This is a really tasty winter warming soup, and another one that can be frozen before you add the yoghurt.

Ingredients

2 tsp coconut oil
1 medium onion, chopped
350g sweet potato, roughly chopped
1 tsp mild curry powder
600–700ml boiling water
1 tsp vegetable bouillon powder
black pepper
1 tbsp 0% fat natural Greek-style yoghurt (optional)

Heat the coconut oil in a saucepan over a medium heat. Once it's hot, add the onion and fry for 5 minutes until softened. Stir in the sweet potato and curry powder and stir for a minute then pour in 600ml of the boiling water and add the bouillon powder and some pepper. Bring to a boil then part cover the pan with a lid and simmer for 20 minutes until the potato is really soft.

Use a stick blender to blitz it smooth, adding a splash more boiling water if needed until you get the consistency you like, but keeping it quite thick.

Spoon the soup into bowls and serve straight away with an optional spoonful of yoghurt on top.

TIP: You can leave the skin on the sweet potatoes for extra goodness, or peel them if you prefer.

Vegetable soup

Serves 2–3

Ingredients

1 tsp coconut oil
1 small onion, chopped
2 sticks celery, chopped
450g root vegetables (carrots, sweet potatoes, parsnips), peeled and diced
1 tsp ground turmeric
750ml boiling water
1 tsp vegetable bouillon powder
50g savoy cabbage or spring greens, shredded
black pepper

VARIATION

Add a drained tin of butter beans, haricot beans or cannellini beans to turn it into a stew for dinner.

You can keep this soup in the fridge for two days and it can also be frozen, so it's a great standby.

Heat the coconut oil in a saucepan over a medium heat. Once it's hot, add the onion and celery and fry for 5 minutes until golden.

Stir in the root vegetables and turmeric then pour in the boiling water and add the bouillon powder. Stir then part cover the pan with a lid, and leave to bubble gently over a medium heat for 15 minutes.

Add the cabbage, put the lid fully on the pan and cook for a further 5 minutes, by which time the root vegetables should be soft. Add some black pepper and serve.

L

Greek salad

Serves 1

Greek salad is one of my all-time favourites since spending so much time in Greece filming *Geordie Shore*. I'm addicted to it!

Ingredients
30g salad leaves
30g feta cheese, crumbled
25g pitted black olives
1 medium tomato, cut into 8 wedges
½ small red onion, thinly sliced
¼ cucumber, diced
black pepper
1 tsp balsamic vinegar

Put the salad leaves on a plate and top with all the other ingredients, finishing with some black pepper and a drizzle of balsamic vinegar.

Serve with a slice of rye bread.

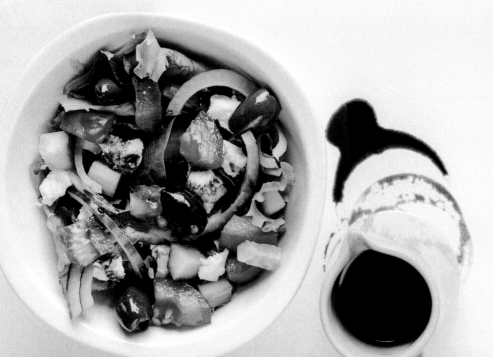

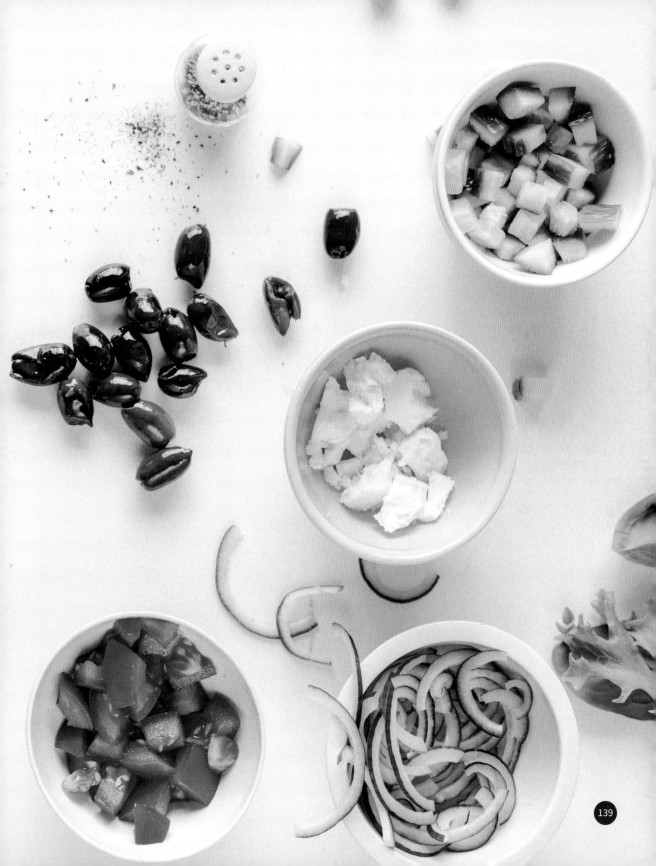

Chicken, mozzarella and tomato salad with pesto

Serves 1

I love mozzarella – cheese is my most favourite thing in the whole world – so having a cheese salad makes me very excited.

Ingredients
35g baby spinach
50–75g ready-cooked skinless chicken breast, thinly sliced or shredded
35g mozzarella, thinly sliced
1 large tomato, thinly sliced
1 tsp ready-made green pesto
a handful of fresh basil leaves (optional)
1 tsp boiling water
salt and black pepper

Scatter the spinach on a plate then top with the slices of chicken, mozzarella and tomato. Season with salt and pepper.

In a small bowl mix the pesto with the boiling water then spoon this over the salad. Tear over the fresh basil leaves, if using, and serve.

VARIATION

This is also good with half a ripe avocado sliced on top.

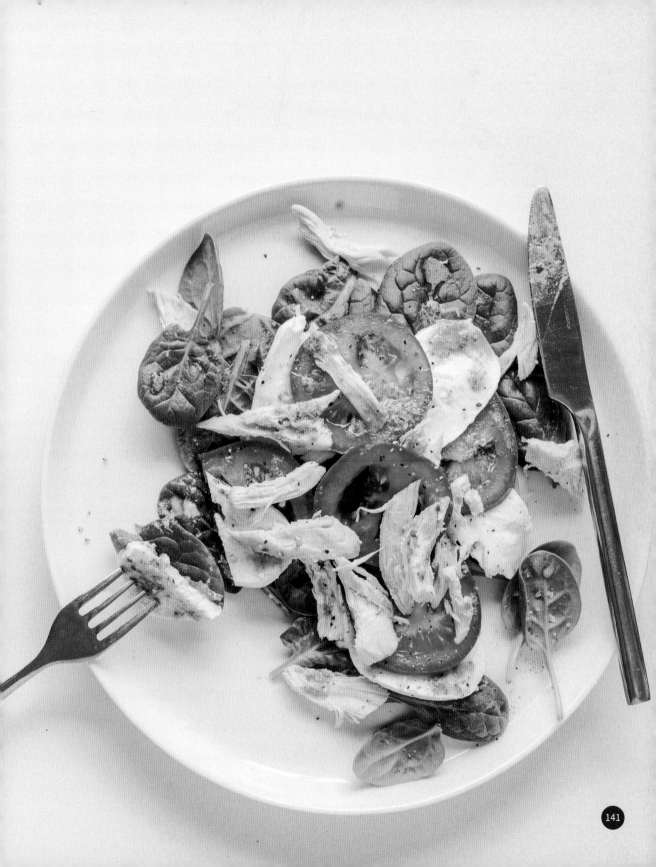

Grilled goats' cheese and sweet potato mash

Serves 1

The tangy flavour of the goats' cheese really transforms the mash, and makes this a lunch in its own right.

Ingredients

250–300g sweet potato, roughly chopped
2 tbsp unsweetened almond milk, oat milk or semi-skimmed milk
40g soft or crumbly goats' cheese, sliced or crumbled depending on type
salt and black pepper

Preheat the grill to medium-high. Boil the sweet potato in a saucepan of boiling, salted water over a medium-high heat for 15 minutes until tender. Drain thoroughly and mash with the milk and some salt and pepper.

Spoon the sweet potato mash into a heatproof dish. Top with the goats' cheese and place under the grill for 5 minutes until bubbling and golden.

Serve on its own, or with a big salad of baby spinach and rocket dressed with a drizzle of balsamic vinegar.

Egg, avocado and rocket salad

Serves 1

Another really easy salad – honestly there's no excuse for not being good.

Ingredients
2 medium free-range eggs
2 tsp hummus
½ tsp Dijon mustard
2 tsp boiling water
35g rocket
1 ripe avocado
black pepper

VARIATION

You can also use watercress or baby spinach in place of the rocket, or a mixture of any of these.

Put a saucepan of water on to boil. Once boiling turn the heat to medium so the water is gently bubbling. Use a spoon to carefully lower in the eggs and boil for 7–8 minutes. Remove from the heat, pour off the water then fill the saucepan with cold water and leave the eggs to cool for a few minutes.

Whisk the hummus, mustard and boiling water together with a fork to make a dressing.

Fill a bowl with the rocket. Peel the eggs, cut them in half and put on top of the salad. Cut the avocado in half, remove the stone and peel away the skin or scoop out the flesh using a spoon. Slice the flesh and scatter around the egg.

Drizzle over the dressing. Add a bit of black pepper and serve.

Goats' cheese, spinach and red pepper frittata

Serves 2–3

You can have this hot one day and cold the next as a packed lunch.

Ingredients

2 tsp coconut oil
1 small red pepper, seeds removed, diced
½ red onion, chopped
50g spinach or baby spinach
6 medium free-range eggs
salt and black pepper
30g soft or crumbly goats' cheese

Preheat the grill to medium high.

Heat half the coconut oil in a non-stick frying pan over a medium heat. Once it's hot, add the red pepper and onion and fry for 2–3 minutes to soften slightly then add the spinach and cook for a minute until it wilts. Scrape the vegetables into a bowl.

Add the remaining coconut oil to the pan. Crack the eggs into a mixing bowl and lightly beat them with a fork with a pinch of salt and some pepper. Pour them into the pan and leave to cook over a medium heat for 3–4 minutes until set on the bottom and still wet on top. Scatter the cooked vegetables and goats' cheese on top.

To finish cooking the frittata pop it under the medium-high grill for 1–2 minutes until golden and bubbling.

Serve hot or cold. Have a big salad on the side, if you like, dressed with a drizzle of balsamic vinegar. Keep any leftovers in the fridge.

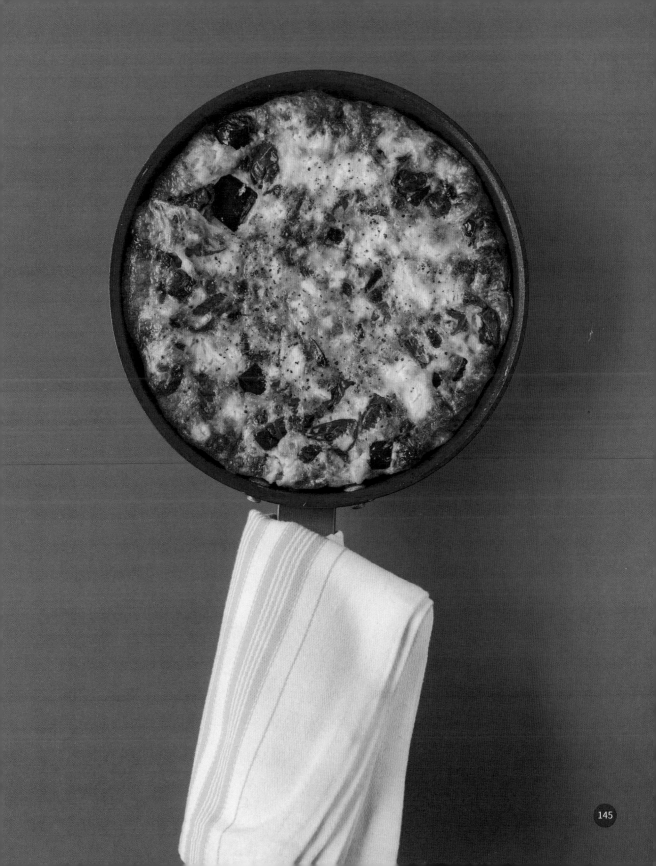

Chickpea, chorizo and spinach soup

Serves 2

This keeps fine in the fridge for two days, so it's good to make a double quantity like this.

Heat the olive oil in a saucepan over a medium heat. Once it's hot, add the chorizo, onion and celery and fry for 5 minutes.

Add the tomatoes then fill the empty tin with water and add to the pan. Stir in the chickpeas and bouillon powder and simmer for 10 minutes.

Stir in the spinach and cook for 1–2 minutes until wilted. Add some black pepper and serve.

Ingredients
1 tsp olive oil
50g cooking chorizo or cured chorizo, finely chopped
1 small onion, chopped
2 sticks celery, chopped
400g tin chopped tomatoes
400g tin chickpeas, drained and rinsed
1 tsp vegetable bouillon powder
100g spinach or baby spinach
black pepper

VARIATION

You can also use cannellini beans, butter beans or haricot beans instead of chickpeas. For a veggie version leave out the chorizo and add 1 teaspoon of sweet smoked paprika.

SEE TIP ON PAGE 104

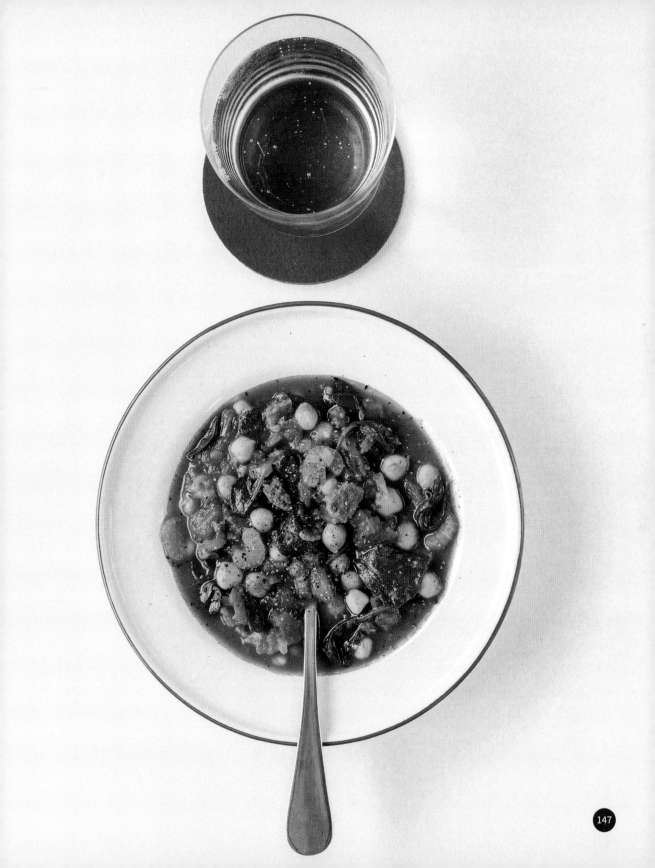

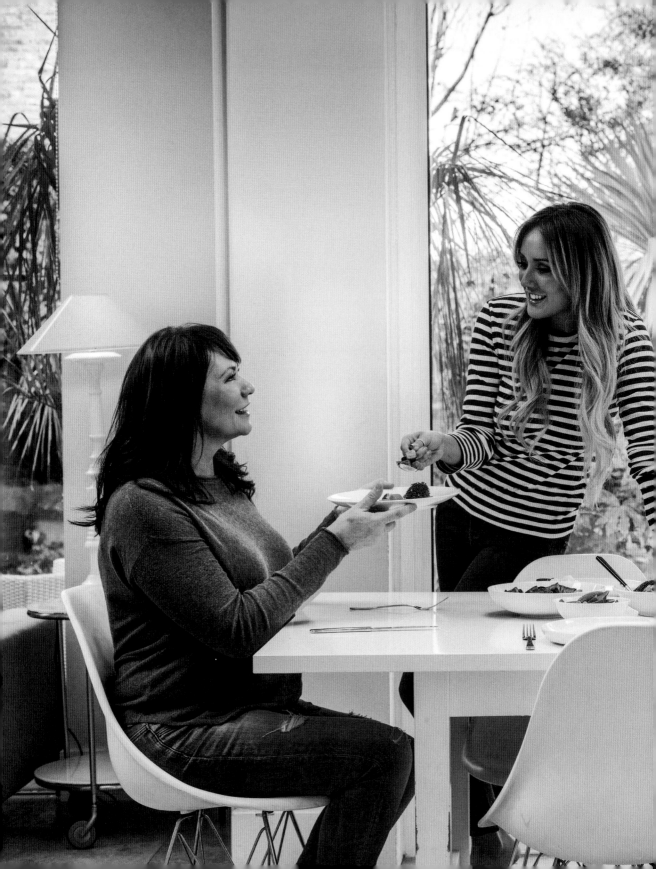

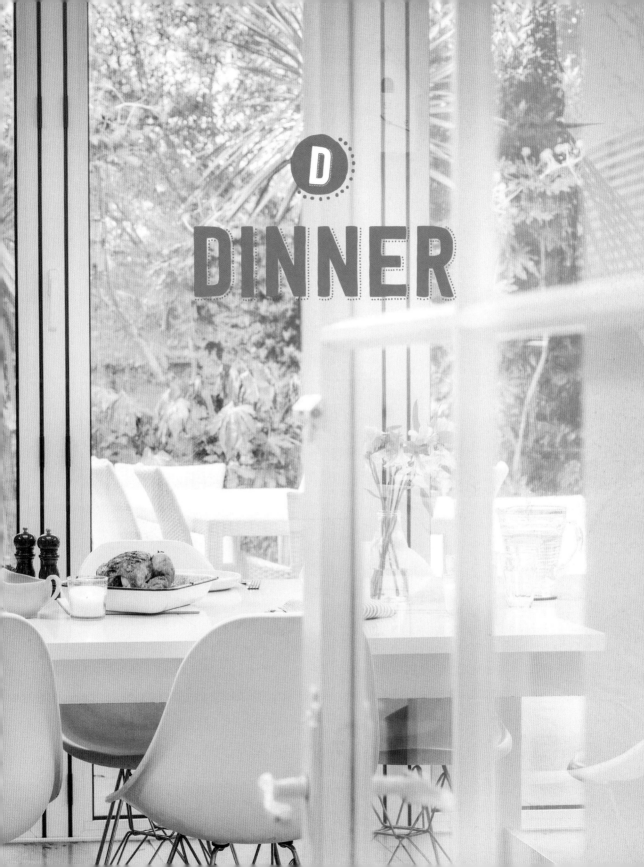

DINNER

Chicken fajitas in lettuce leaves

Serves 2

I love chicken fajitas, they used to be mine and Mitch's favourite dish. These are practically the same but without the wraps – I prefer them now.

Ingredients

1 tsp coconut oil
1 red pepper, seeds removed, thinly sliced
1 medium onion, thinly sliced
2 boneless and skinless chicken breasts, cut into strips
1 heaped tsp fajita seasoning or piri piri spice blend
1 ripe avocado
25g feta or crumbly goats' cheese, crumbled
4 tbsp 0% fat natural Greek-style yoghurt
1 lime, cut into wedges (optional)
8 lettuce leaves from a crisp lettuce (e.g. little gem, iceberg or romaine)

For the chicken, heat the coconut oil in a large, non-stick frying pan or wok over a high heat. Add the red pepper and onion and fry, stirring often, for 2–3 minutes, then add the chicken and the fajita seasoning and fry for 6–7 minutes, stirring often, or until the chicken is completely cooked through. Turn off the heat and leave in the pan.

To assemble, cut the avocado in half, remove the stone then peel away the skin or scoop out the flesh with a spoon. Cut into slices and put in a bowl. Fill a small bowl or ramekin with the cheese, another with the yoghurt and a third with the lime wedges, if using.

Divide the lettuce leaves between two plates. Using the lettuce leaves as if they were wraps, put some of the hot chicken and red pepper mixture in one of the lettuce leaves and top with some of the cheese, yoghurt, avocado and a squeeze of lime, if using. Roll up the leaves to encase the filling and eat with your fingers! Repeat with the rest of the chicken and lettuce leaves.

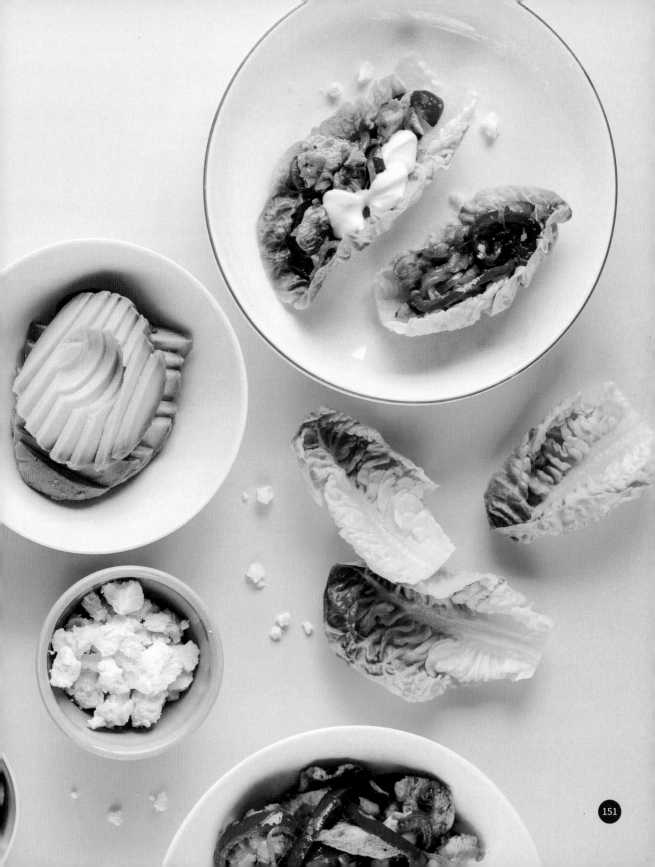

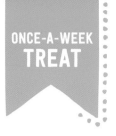

Steak with mustard, onion and mushrooms

Serves 2

It's good to have protein when you can and this is a nice one for an evening meal to fill you up. I use a George Foreman electric grill, so I just rub the ingredients with some of the coconut oil before grilling.

Ingredients

3 tsp coconut oil
4 Portobello mushrooms, stalks trimmed
1 onion, thinly sliced
2 sirloin steaks, each weighing about 150g, excess fat trimmed
2 tsp Dijon or wholegrain mustard
80g savoy cabbage, spring greens or cabbage, chopped
1 red chilli, finely chopped (optional)
salt and black pepper

VARIATION

Instead of the stir-fried cabbage you can serve this with steamed or boiled broccoli if you prefer.

Preheat the oven to 75ºC and put two heatproof plates in to warm.

Heat 2 teaspoons of the coconut oil in a non-stick frying pan over a medium-high heat. Add the mushrooms, stalk side down, and scatter the onion alongside. Place a small pan lid directly onto the mushrooms to weigh them down. Cook for 5–6 minutes, turning halfway, then transfer to the warm plates and keep warm in the oven.

Season the steaks on both sides with salt and pepper. Add the rest of the coconut oil to the pan and fry the steaks for 2 minutes on each side (or 3–4 minutes for well done). Remove from the pan, smear with the mustard and keep warm with the mushrooms and onion.

Add the cabbage and chilli to the steak pan and stir-fry over a medium-high heat for 2–3 minutes. Serve with the steak, mushrooms and onion.

TIP: If you have a large enough frying pan you can cook the mushrooms, onion and steak all at the same time.

Healthy meatballs with pepper sauce

Serves 2

I love having healthy meatballs – this is great for a date night meal.

Ingredients

1 small red pepper, seeds removed, roughly chopped
1 small yellow pepper, seeds removed, roughly chopped
400g tin chopped tomatoes
½ tsp chilli powder or paprika
1½ tsp balsamic vinegar (optional)
200g lean minced beef (less than 5% fat if you can get it)
½ medium red onion, finely chopped
½ tbsp coconut oil
35g baby spinach
40g feta cheese, crumbled
salt and black pepper

For the sauce, use a stick blender or liquidiser to blitz the peppers with the tomatoes, chilli powder, balsamic vinegar, if using, and a pinch of salt until smooth. Set aside.

Using clean hands mix the beef and onion together with a pinch of salt and pepper. Divide into eight and roll into balls. Heat the coconut oil in a non-stick frying pan over a medium heat. Add the meatballs and fry, turning regularly, for 5–6 minutes or until brown all over.

Add the tomato sauce to the pan. Once it's bubbling turn down the heat to low and cover the pan with a lid. Cook for 10 minutes. Stir in the spinach leaves for a minute until wilted then crumble over the feta cheese.

Serve the meatballs in their sauce with brown rice and Tenderstem or regular broccoli.

TIP: To save time you can buy ready-rolled, raw meatballs in most supermarkets, although they will probably be higher in fat.

Lower-fat burger with Portobello bun and sweet potato fries

Serves 2

Ingredients

400g sweet potato, cut into chips
2 tsp fajita seasoning or
piri piri spice blend
2 medium free-range eggs
250g lean minced beef (less than
5% fat if you can get it)
½ medium red onion, finely chopped
2 tsp coconut oil
4 large Portobello mushrooms,
stalks trimmed
lettuce leaves
1 medium tomato, sliced
½ medium red onion, cut into rings
black pepper

Seeing as I was addicted to fast food and especially burgers, I'm over the moon that I still get to eat them.

Preheat the oven to 200°C/gas 6. For the sweet potato fries, toss the sweet potato, spice mix and some pepper together in a non-stick roasting tin. Crack the eggs into a bowl, lightly beat, then mix with the sweet potato. Cook in the oven for 40 minutes.

While they're cooking, get going with the burgers. Mix the mince, onion and pepper together with your hands and shape into two burgers.

Heat 1 teaspoon of the coconut oil in a non-stick frying pan over a medium heat. When hot add the burgers and fry for 7 minutes on each side, or until cooked through.

While the burgers are cooking, place the mushrooms stalk side down on a baking tray, top each with a ½ teaspoon of coconut oil and cook in the oven for 10 minutes. Turn them over and cook for a further 5 minutes until softened and browned.

Put each burger on top of one of the mushrooms, add the lettuce, tomato slices and onion rings, then place the second mushroom on top like a bun. Serve with the sweet potato fries.

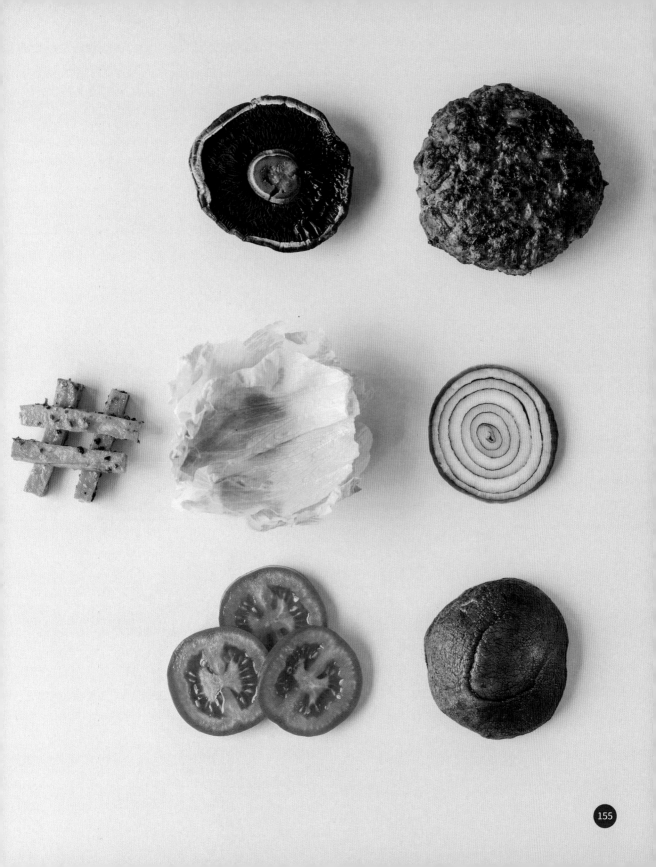

Piri piri chicken with roast sweet potatoes

Serves 2

Who doesn't love a cheeky Nando's? This is how I do it at home.

Ingredients

2 tbsp lemon juice, or juice of 1 lemon
2 tsp piri piri spice mix
2 tsp coconut oil
2 boneless and skinless chicken breasts
400g medium sweet potatoes, cut into bite-sized chunks
100g cherry tomatoes, halved
salt and black pepper

Preheat the oven to 200°C/gas 6. Mix the lemon juice and piri piri in a shallow bowl. Add the chicken breasts to the bowl. Prick the chicken all over with a fork and toss to coat in the mixture. Set aside.

Put the coconut oil in a large, non-stick roasting tin and put in the oven for a minute, or until it has melted. Add the sweet potato with some salt and pepper and toss to coat in the oil. Roast in the oven for 20 minutes.

Scatter the tomatoes into the roasting tin and stir into the potatoes. Make a gap in the middle and put the chicken breasts in the gap. Pour the piri piri and lemon juice mixture mainly over the chicken, drizzling a little over the tomatoes and sweet potato. Roast in the oven for another 20 minutes, or until the chicken is completely cooked through.

Serve the chicken and roast sweet potatoes with some Tenderstem or regular broccoli alongside.

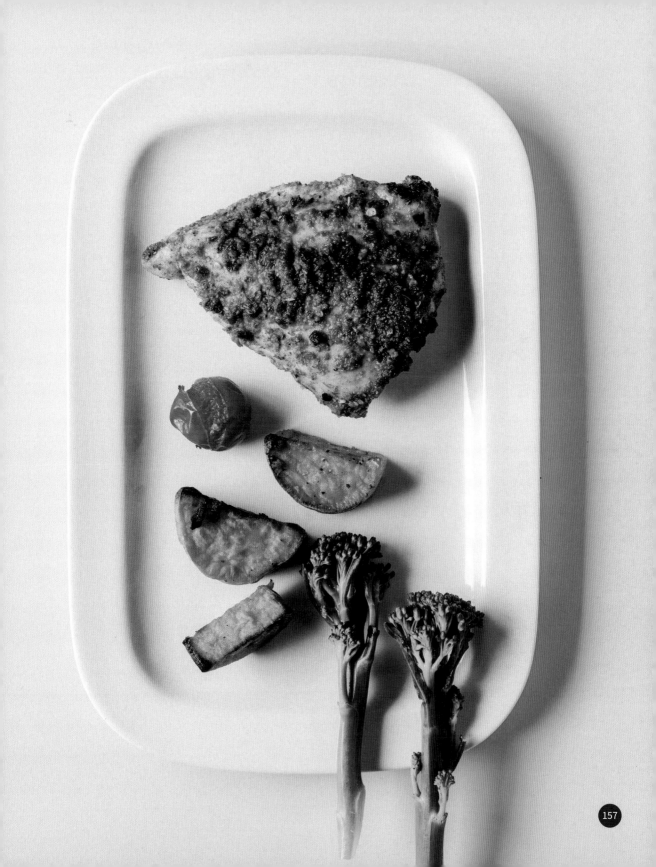

One-pan roast garlic chicken

Serves 2

So juicy, so tasty. Just remember to give your teeth a clean afterwards.

Ingredients

2 boneless and skinless chicken breasts
125g mushrooms, left whole
1 medium onion, cut into 8 wedges
1 apple, cut into 8 wedges and cored
4 cloves garlic, peeled and left whole
1 tsp dried mixed herbs or dried tarragon
2 tsp wholegrain mustard
1 tsp coconut oil
1 tsp vegetable bouillon powder mixed with 50ml boiling water
black pepper

Preheat the oven to 180°C/gas 4.

Place the chicken breasts in the middle of a non-stick roasting tin and scatter the mushrooms, onion, apple and garlic around them.

Season everything with pepper, and sprinkle over the dried herbs. Rub the wholegrain mustard and coconut oil over the chicken breasts.

Pour the bouillon powder mixed with the boiling water into the roasting tin then cover the tin tightly with foil. Cook in the oven for 25 minutes, or until the vegetables are tender and the chicken is cooked through.

Spoon the juices over the chicken and vegetables. Serve with some steamed green veg on the side.

TIP: You can also cook this in a roasting bag to help keep the chicken extra moist during cooking.

Cottage pie with sweet potato topping

Serves 2–3

Ingredients

2 tsp coconut oil
1 medium onion, chopped
1 clove garlic, peeled and
finely chopped
250g lean minced beef (less than 5%
fat if you can get it)
1 heaped tsp dried mixed herbs
1 medium carrot, chopped or
coarsely grated
75g mushrooms, chopped
400g tin chopped tomatoes
2 medium sweet potatoes (350g), cut
into chunks
2 heaped tbsp 0% fat natural
Greek-style yoghurt
2 tbsp unsweetened almond milk,
oat milk or semi-skimmed milk
salt and black pepper

Mmm… This one is perfect for a cold day. It'll warm up your cockles and keep you satisfied for hours.

Preheat the oven to 200°C/gas 6.

For the filling, heat the coconut oil in a large, non-stick frying pan over a medium heat, add the onion and fry for 5 minutes, then stir in the garlic and fry for another minute. Add the mince, turn the heat up to medium-high and fry the mince, breaking up any big lumps, for 5 minutes or until browned, then stir in the herbs, carrot and mushrooms and fry for 3 minutes.

Add the tomatoes. Half-fill the empty tin with water and add this to the pan. Season with salt and pepper before putting a lid on the pan. Simmer over a medium-low heat for 30 minutes. While the filling is cooking, boil the sweet potato in a pan of boiling water with a pinch of salt for 15 minutes or until tender. Drain well and mash with the yoghurt and milk.

Spoon the filling into a baking dish (roughly 20-cm square), top with the sweet potato mash, draw lines on top with a fork and cook in the oven, on a baking tray, for 15–20 minutes until golden brown and bubbling.

Serve the cottage pie with steamed spring greens.

Healthy roast dinner

Serves 4

I love Sunday dinners. I'd never like to cut them out of my life, that's why this healthy one is a lifesaver. Make sure you just have a small bit of the meat – and fill up with loads of veg.

Ingredients

2 medium onions, sliced
1 lemon, sliced
1 whole chicken weighing 1.2–1.4kg
1 tbsp coconut oil, plus 1 tsp for the gravy
700g sweet potatoes, peeled and cut into bite-sized chunks
1 tsp chilli powder or paprika
300ml boiling water
1½ tsp vegetable bouillon powder
2 tsp cornflour
2 tbsp apple juice
½ tsp balsamic vinegar
2 medium carrots, cut into 1cm-thick rounds
200g broccoli, cut into small florets
200g cauliflower, cut into small florets
150g green beans, mangetout or sugar snaps, trimmed and halved
100g frozen peas
salt and black pepper

Preheat the oven to 200°C/gas 6. For the roast chicken, spread half the sliced onion and the lemon slices in a small non-stick roasting tin. Put the chicken on top, breast side down. Season with salt and pepper and pour 4 tablespoons of water into the tin. Roast for 30 minutes then turn the chicken over, spoon over the juices and roast for a further 20–30 minutes. Add a splash of boiling water if needed to keep the onion moist.

While the chicken is cooking, put 1 tablespoon of coconut oil in a large non-stick roasting tin and melt in the oven for 2–3 minutes. Tip the sweet potato into the tin, sprinkle with the chilli powder, salt and pepper and stir around to coat thoroughly in the oil. Roast for 30–40 minutes in the oven with the chicken, stirring halfway, until tender and browned at the edges.

Make the gravy while the chicken and potato are roasting. Heat 1 teaspoon of coconut oil in a saucepan over a medium heat. Add the remaining onion and fry for 10 minutes until softened and golden. Pour in the boiling

Cont...

water and the bouillon powder and bring to a boil. Boil for 2–3 minutes then turn off the heat.

In a small bowl, mix the cornflour with the apple juice until smooth, then stir this into the gravy. Return the pan to a low heat and stir for 2–3 minutes until thickened. Stir in the balsamic vinegar and season with lots of black pepper. Keep warm on a low heat. If the gravy gets too thick add a splash of boiling water.

Remove the chicken from the oven. To check the chicken is cooked pierce the thickest part of the thigh with a sharp knife and check the juices run clear (there should be no blood or pink juices). Also test that the legs pull away easily from the body. Let it rest for 5–10 minutes before carving (this makes the chicken juicier).

While the chicken is resting bring a large pan of salted water to the boil. Add the carrots and cook for 3 minutes then add the rest of the veggies and cook for 3–4 minutes until tender but still crisp. Drain thoroughly.

Serve a bit of everything on warm plates.

TIP: To save time you can use a bag of frozen mixed veggies to replace the mound of veg in the recipe.

Lamb chops with mounds of roasted veg

Serves 2

Ingredients

4 lamb chops, each weighing around 100g, excess fat trimmed
1 heaped tbsp coconut oil
1 medium red onion, cut into wedges
1 yellow pepper, seeds removed, cut into bite-sized chunks
1 red pepper, seeds removed, cut into bite-sized chunks
1 aubergine, seeds removed, cut into bite-sized chunks
200g sweet potatoes, cut into bite-sized chunks
1 courgette, sliced into 1cm-thick rounds
2 large tomatoes, cut into quarters
½ tsp dried oregano or dried, mixed herbs
salt and black pepper

As lamb's a bit fattier than other meats, try to avoid any other fatty foods on a day you have this for dinner.

Preheat the oven to 200°C/gas 6.

Season the lamb chops with black pepper and place on a baking tray. Set aside so they come to room temperature while you get on with the veg (this makes the chops juicier).

For the roasted veg, put the coconut oil in a large non-stick roasting tin and heat it in the oven for a minute or until it has melted. Tip all of the prepared veg into the roasting tin, sprinkle with the oregano or mixed herbs and a ½ teaspoon of salt and stir thoroughly to coat the veg with the oil. Put the tin in the oven.

When the veg have been roasting for 20 minutes stir them and return them to the oven at the same time as putting the lamb chops in the oven. Cook for 20 minutes.

Remove the lamb chops from the oven and serve on warmed plates with the roasted veg alongside.

Veggie stew with butter beans

Serves 2

This stew is a great vegetarian dinner and a way of having some protein without eating any meat.

Ingredients

2 tsp coconut oil
1 medium red onion, sliced
2 courgettes, halved lengthways and sliced into 1cm half moons
2 red peppers, seeds removed, halved and sliced
400g tin chopped tomatoes
400g tin butter beans, drained and rinsed
1 tsp sweet smoked paprika
200g spinach or baby spinach
salt and black pepper

VARIATION

For a meaty version, dice a raw boneless and skinless chicken breast and add along with the courgettes and peppers. For a fishy version, drain a tin of tuna in brine and stir in with the spinach.

Heat the coconut oil in a saucepan or flameproof casserole over a medium heat. Once it's hot, add the onion and fry for 5 minutes until softened. Stir in the courgettes and red peppers and fry for 5 minutes, then stir in the tomatoes, butter beans and paprika. Half-fill the empty tomato tin with water and pour into the stew. Add the sweet smoked paprika, salt and pepper and simmer, part covered, for 20 minutes.

Give everything a good mix then stir in the spinach, put the lid back on and cook for 3–4 minutes (it will seem like a lot of spinach but it will shrink right down when cooked), adding a splash more water if needed.

Spoon into bowls and serve.

Chicken and prawn stir-fry

Serves 2

Another meal inspired by my love of a takeaway –
I just can't get enough of Chinese food.

Ingredients

100g dried rice noodles
2 tsp coconut oil
1 boneless and skinless chicken breast, cut into strips
1 large clove garlic, peeled and finely chopped
4-cm piece root ginger, peeled and finely grated
1 red chilli, sliced
150g raw king prawns, defrosted if frozen
1 medium red onion, sliced
1 red, orange or yellow pepper, seeds removed, thinly sliced
50g frozen peas
1 medium carrot, coarsely grated
2 tsp dark soy sauce or tamari
black pepper

Cook the noodles according to the packet instructions.

Place a wok or large non-stick frying pan on a medium-high heat. Add the coconut oil. When hot, add the chicken, garlic, ginger and chilli, stir-frying for 5–6 minutes until the chicken is browned and cooked through.

Add the prawns and stir-fry for 3 minutes, or until completely pink, then add the vegetables and fry for 2 more minutes. Add the soy sauce and black pepper and mix well. Toss the noodles through the stir-fry.

Serve on warmed plates or in bowls.

TIP: When cooking a stir-fry it's a good idea to have all the ingredients prepared and next to the hob as everything's needed quickly. Or to save time chopping, substitute the vegetables for 250g pre-prepared stir-fry veg.

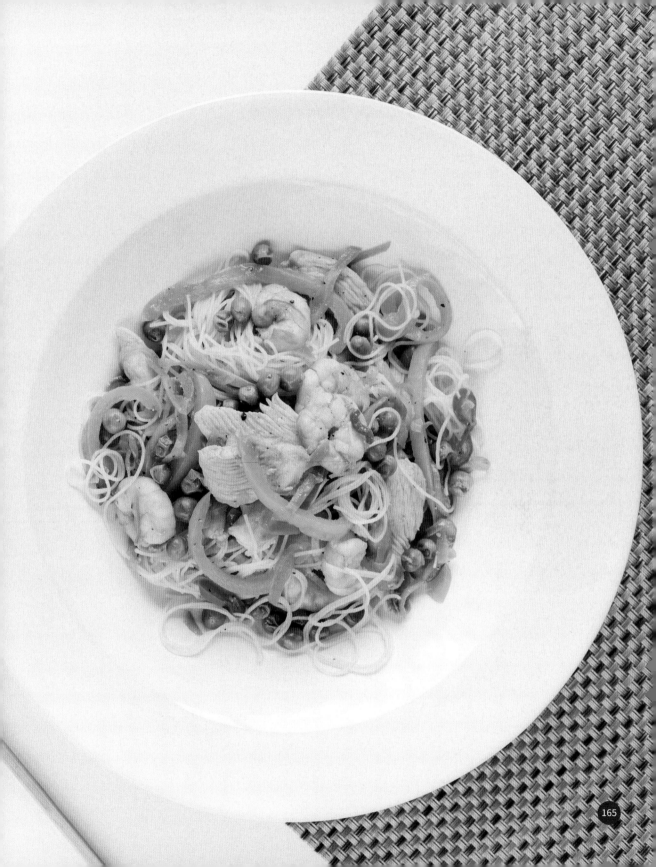

Teriyaki salmon with ginger and broccoli

Serves 2

Ingredients

150g Tenderstem broccoli, halved
lengthways if stalks are thick, or
green beans
2 chunky salmon fillets, each
weighing 125–150g, skin on
4-cm piece root ginger, peeled and
thinly sliced
1 clove garlic, peeled and
thinly sliced
1 tbsp dark soy sauce or tamari
4 tbsp water
black pepper
½ lime, cut in half
4 spring onions, trimmed and
finely sliced

This a really tasty variation on my favourite fish.

Preheat the oven to 220°C/gas 7. Tear two pieces of tin foil, each roughly 30 x 40cm.

Divide the broccoli between the two pieces of foil and arrange in the middle. Put a salmon fillet on top, skin side down, then scatter the garlic and ginger on top of the salmon and drizzle over the soy sauce. Season with black pepper and pour 2 tablespoons of water into each parcel around the broccoli.

Wrap the parcels, scrunching the edges tightly so no steam can escape. Put on a baking tray and cook in the oven for 15–18 minutes.

Carefully unwrap the parcels, squeeze over the lime juice, scatter with the spring onions and serve with the lime wedges.

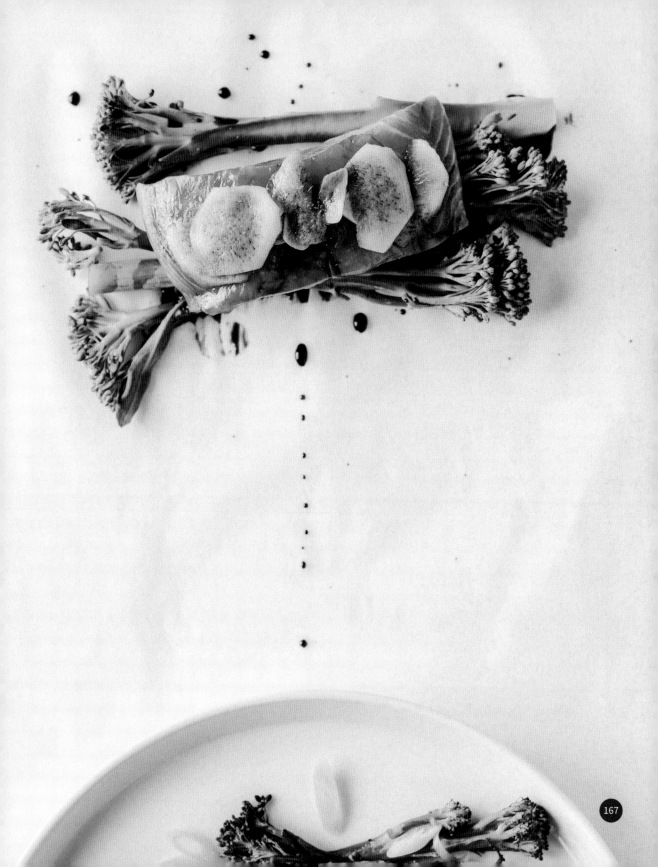

One-pan eggs rancheros

Serves 2

Ingredients

1 tsp coconut oil
1 medium red onion, sliced
2 red peppers, seeds removed, sliced
1 clove garlic, sliced
1 tsp sweet smoked paprika
400g tin chopped tomatoes
100g spinach or baby spinach, washed
6 medium free-range eggs
salt and black pepper

This is one I often have after a day's training.

Heat the coconut oil in a large non-stick frying pan on a medium-high heat. Add the onion and peppers and fry for 5 minutes until softened, then add the garlic and fry for a minute.

Stir in the smoked paprika, salt and pepper, and tomatoes. Half-fill the empty tomato tin with water and pour into the pan. Bubble for 15 minutes over a medium heat until the sauce is thick. Stir in the spinach and cook for 1 minute until wilted.

Crack the first egg into a cup. Make a small gap in the sauce and use the cup to gently lower the egg into the gap. Repeat with the remaining eggs. Season the eggs with a pinch of salt and pepper.

Cover the pan with a lid or a baking tray and cook for 3–4 minutes or until cooked to your liking. Use a wooden or plastic spatula to remove the eggs rancheros to two plates to serve.

TIP: You could also finish this under the grill.

Sweet potato and chickpea curry with spinach

Serves 2

This curry is bloody amazing, and filling enough to have it without rice if you prefer.

Ingredients

2 tsp coconut oil
1 medium red onion, sliced
1 clove garlic, peeled and sliced
3 tsp ground cumin
1½ tsp turmeric
1 tsp chilli powder or paprika
400g sweet potatoes, cut into bite-sized pieces
400ml boiling water
1 tsp vegetable bouillon powder
400g tin chickpeas, drained and rinsed
200g spinach or baby spinach
½ lime, cut into wedges
salt and black pepper

VARIATION

For a tomato version, replace the water and stock with a 400g tin of chopped tomatoes and replace the spices with 1 heaped teaspoon of smoked paprika.

Heat the coconut oil in a saucepan or flameproof casserole over a medium heat. Once it's hot, add the onion and fry for 5 minutes until softened. Stir in the garlic and fry for a minute then stir in the cumin, turmeric and chilli, followed by the sweet potato.

Give the sweet potato a good stir then pour in 300ml of the boiling water and the bouillon powder and stir, scraping up any browned bits from the bottom of the pan. Bring to a simmer, cover with a lid and cook over a medium heat for 10 minutes. Add a splash more boiling water if it gets too dry.

Stir in the chickpeas, cover the pan and cook for another 10 minutes until the sweet potato is tender. Stir in the spinach, put the lid back on and cook for 2–3 minutes until the spinach has just wilted but is still bright green. Add a bit of salt and pepper if needed.

Serve with lime wedges and a small portion of brown rice.

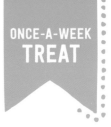

ONCE-A-WEEK TREAT

Mushroom and chicken pie

Serves 2

Who doesn't love a good old pie?

Ingredients

300g boneless and skinless chicken thighs
salt and black pepper
2 tsp coconut oil, plus 1 tsp extra for greasing
500g brown mushrooms
2 cloves garlic, peeled
1 tbsp cornflour, mixed to a paste with 1 tbsp of cold water
400ml hot chicken stock (fresh or made from a good-quality stock cube)
4–6 sheets filo pastry

VARIATION

For a real comforting treat you could serve this with a half-portion of the Root veg mash on page 180.

Preheat the oven to 180°C/gas 4.

Lay the chicken thighs flat and season with salt and pepper. Heat a medium non-stick frying pan over a medium-high heat and melt the coconut oil. Add the chicken and fry for 5 minutes on one side until lightly browned, then turn over and cook for a further 5 minutes. Remove to a plate, cover with foil and leave while you make the sauce.

Blitz the mushrooms and garlic cloves in a food processor until finely chopped (or finely chop by hand) and add to the same pan used to cook the chicken. Stir over a medium-high heat for 6–8 minutes, or until the water has evaporated from the mushrooms. Reduce the heat to medium.

Shred or chop the chicken and add it to the pan with the mushrooms along with any juice on the plate. Stir in the cornflour paste and stock and cook for 5 minutes, then spoon into a round or oval pie dish, about 23cm in diameter. Rub the remaining teaspoon of coconut oil lightly between your palms then lightly scrunch each filo pastry sheet to coat it in the oil and place them on top of the filling.

Place the pie dish on a baking tray and cook for 15 minutes until the filling is bubbling and the pastry golden. Serve the pie piping hot with green vegetables.

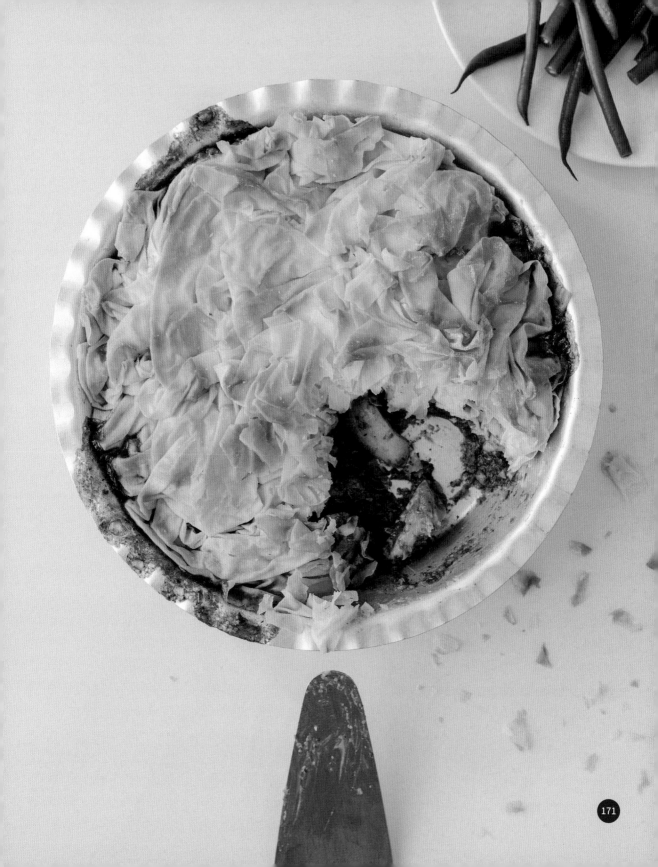

Cod with chorizo, red peppers, onion and tomatoes

Serves 2

I try to have lots of fish in my diet and this is a great recipe for cod.

Ingredients

2 tsp olive oil
25g cooking chorizo or cured chorizo, finely chopped
1 medium red onion, sliced
1 large red pepper, seeds removed, thinly sliced
400g tin chopped tomatoes
2 fillets of cod loin, each weighing around 150g
salt and black pepper

VARIATION

You can use any firm white fish, so haddock, pollock and hake all work well.

Heat the olive oil in a non-stick frying pan over a medium-high heat. Once it's hot, add the chorizo, onion and red pepper and fry for 5 minutes until the onion is just turning golden. Add the tomatoes and some salt and pepper. Quarter-fill the empty tomato tin with water, swirl it round, and add to the pan.

Once the sauce is bubbling add the cod and season the top of the fish with salt and pepper. Reduce the heat to medium, cook for 3 minutes then carefully turn the cod over and cook for 10 more minutes or until the fish is cooked through (cut into the thickest part and it should be an opaque white all the way through).

Serve the cod with the sauce spooned over it and a big portion of streamed green veg on the side.

Spicy lamb stew with garlic sweet potato mash

Serves 2

Ingredients

250g lamb leg steak, excess fat
trimmed, cut into small pieces
1 medium red onion, thinly sliced
400g tin chickpeas, drained
and rinsed
½ 400g tin chopped tomatoes
500ml hot chicken stock or
vegetable stock
½ tsp ras-el-hanout spice blend or
piri piri spice blend
100g green beans, cut into
bite-sized lengths
350g sweet potatoes, peeled and
roughly chopped
1 fresh red chili, cut in half lengthwise
(optional)
1 clove garlic, left in the skin
(optional)
salt and black pepper

**I know lamb is quite a fatty meat, but you are
allowed to have fat in moderation.**

For the stew add the lamb, onion, chickpeas, tomatoes,
stock and spice blend to a flameproof casserole or
heavy frying pan (with a tightly fitting lid) and bring to a
boil, then cover and cook on a low heat for 40 minutes,
stirring occasionally and adding the green beans for the
last 4 minutes.

When the stew has been in the oven for 20 minutes, boil
the sweet potato, chilli and garlic, if using, in a saucepan
of boiling, salted water over a medium-high heat for
10–15 minutes until just tender but not mushy. Drain.

Discard the chilli. Squeeze the garlic from its skin and
discard the skin. Mash the potato and garlic.

Season the stew with black pepper and serve with
the mash.

Easy tomato sauce

Serves 2

This is a great thing to have in your fridge for when you need to make a quick and easy meal.

Ingredients
2 tsp olive oil
2 cloves garlic, peeled and thinly sliced
400g tin chopped tomatoes
½ tsp dried mixed herbs or dried oregano (optional)
salt and black pepper

Heat the olive oil in a non-stick frying pan over a medium heat. Add the garlic and fry for a minute until golden and smelling sweet, but be very careful not to let it get too brown or burn.

Stir in the tomatoes and herbs. Quarter-fill the empty tomato tin with water and add to the pan. Cook, bubbling gently, for 10–15 minutes, stirring occasionally. Season with salt and pepper.

TIP: This sauce keeps in the fridge for three days or can be frozen.

Cont...

To make the prepared sauce into a meal for one or two people (depending on appetite) you can:

• Stir in a 200g tin of drained tuna in brine (150g drained weight) and a handful of black olives and cook in the sauce for 2–3 minutes. If you like capers, add 1 tablespoon of drained capers in brine.

• Add a diced red pepper and fry for 3–4 minutes before you add the garlic, then proceed as opposite. At the end, stir in a 200g tin of drained tuna in brine (150g drained weight) and a peeled and quartered hard-boiled egg and cook for 2–3 minutes.

• Stir in a diced, ready-cooked skinless chicken breast and cook in the sauce for 3–4 minutes until piping hot, then stir in a big handful of baby spinach so it wilts.

• Before adding the garlic, fry a diced onion, a diced red, yellow or orange pepper and a diced courgette for 5–6 minutes then add the garlic and proceed as opposite.

• Before adding the garlic, brown 150g of lean minced beef (less than 5% fat) or minced turkey for 5 minutes over a medium-high heat then lower the heat to medium, add the garlic and proceed as opposite.

• Before adding the garlic, fry 75g of chopped mushrooms for 5–6 minutes then add the garlic and proceed as opposite. Stir in 1–2 slices of lean ham (about 50g), diced, at the end and heat through for a minute or two.

Lower-fat beef chilli with guacamole and yoghurt

Serves 2

I love hot, spicy food and chilli is one of my favourites that me mam makes – this is a healthy alternative.

Ingredients

2 tsp coconut oil
1 medium onion, sliced
1 clove garlic, sliced
1 tsp ground cumin
½ tsp hot paprika or chilli powder, or
1 tsp mild chilli powder
250g lean minced beef (less than 5% fat if you can get it)
1 large or 2 small red peppers, seeds removed, sliced
400g tin chopped tomatoes
400g tin kidney beans, drained and rinsed
1 ripe avocado
½ tbsp lime juice, or juice of ½ lime
4 cherry tomatoes, roughly chopped
1 small red onion, finely chopped
½ fresh red chilli, or
¼ tsp chilli powder
2 tbsp 0% fat natural Greek-style yoghurt
a handful of fresh coriander leaves and stalks, roughly chopped
salt and black pepper

For the chilli, heat the coconut oil in a large non-stick frying pan over a medium heat, add the onion and fry for 5 minutes then stir in the garlic and fry for a minute. Add the spices then the mince, turn the heat up to medium-high and fry for 5 minutes, stirring to break up any big lumps of mince.

Add the pepper and tomatoes. Half-fill the empty tin with water and add this to the pan, then season with salt and pepper. Turn the heat to medium-low and simmer, covered, for 20 minutes, stirring occasionally.

Stir in the kidney beans, cover and cook for another 10 minutes.

While the chilli is cooking, make the guacamole. Cut the avocado in half, peel away the skin and mash the flesh in a bowl with the lime juice and a pinch of salt. Mix in the cherry tomatoes, onion and fresh chilli.

Serve the beef chilli on brown rice with the guacamole and yoghurt on the side and coriander sprinkled over.

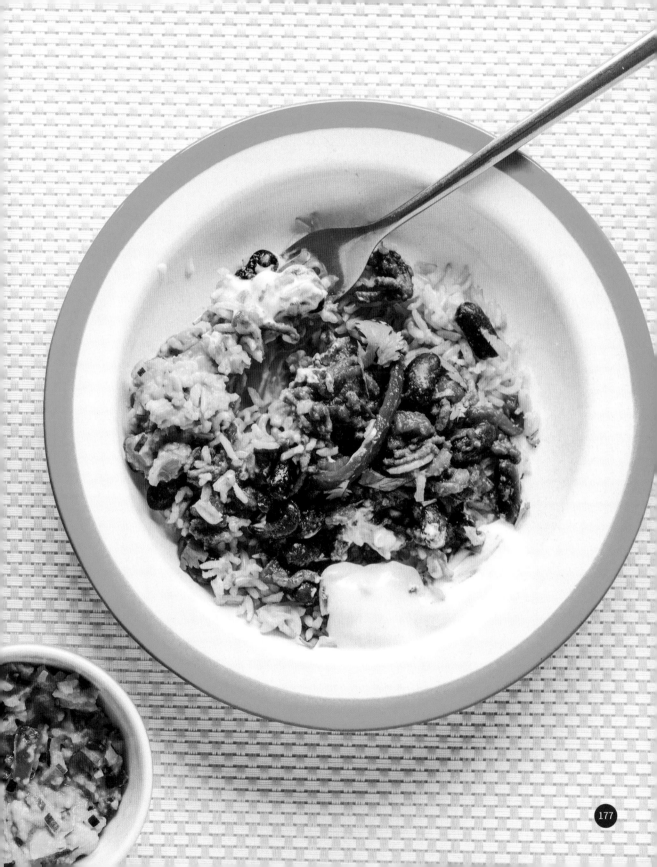

Soy-glazed pork chops with healthy slaw

Serves 2

I don't eat a lot of meat other than chicken, but this pork dish makes a nice change and it's fine to include fattier meats in your diet in moderation.

Ingredients

2 tsp dark soy sauce or tamari
2 tbsp Dijon mustard
2 thick pork chops, each weighing around 200g, excess fat trimmed
1 medium carrot, peeled and coarsely grated
½ medium red onion, thinly sliced
100g white cabbage, shredded
1 green apple, coarsely grated
1 tbsp hummus
few drops of Tabasco sauce (optional)
salt and black pepper

In a small bowl mix the soy sauce and mustard well to combine. Pat the chops dry with kitchen paper and cover them with the mixture. Place into a non-stick roasting tin and season with black pepper and a little salt. Set aside for 15–30 minutes to bring to room temperature. Preheat the oven to 180°C/gas 4.

Put the pork chops in the oven and cook for 30 minutes.

Meanwhile make the slaw by mixing the carrot, onion, cabbage and apple with the hummus and a few drops of Tabasco if you like.

Transfer the chops onto a plate and serve with a mound of slaw alongside.

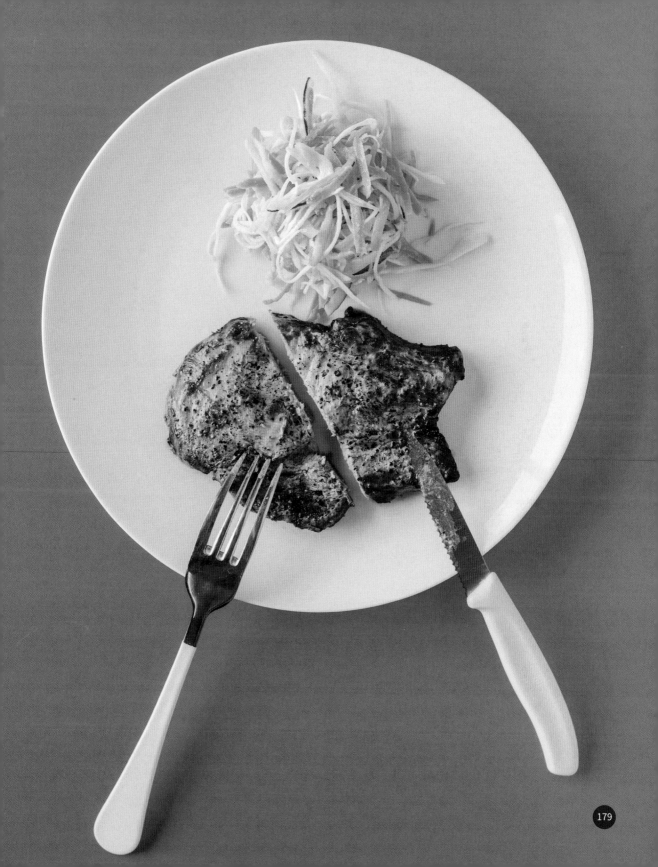

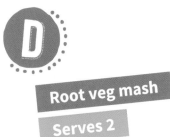

Root veg mash

Serves 2

This mash is great when you're feeling hungry for a bit more than steamed vegetables. It works well with loads of my recipes.

Bring a large pan of salted water to the boil, add all the veg and boil gently over a medium heat for 20–25 minutes or until the vegetables are tender.

Drain thoroughly then mash in the pan with the milk and some black pepper. Serve. The mash keeps in the fridge for two days or can be frozen.

TIP: You can leave the skins on the veg for extra goodness, or peel them if you prefer.

Ingredients

750g root veg (sweet potatoes, carrots, parsnips), cut into small chunks
3 tbsp unsweetened almond milk, oat milk or semi-skimmed milk
salt and black pepper

VARIATION

Eat this on its own with a slice of lean ham or cooked turkey, or serve it as a side dish with Roast lemon and mustard salmon (see page 194) or Cod with chorizo, red peppers, onion (see page 172). As a side dish, these quantities will serve four people.

Easy chicken and veg casserole

Serves 2

Ingredients
500–700ml chicken stock or
vegetable stock
1 medium carrot, roughly chopped
1 medium parsnip, roughly chopped
1½ tbsp wholegrain mustard or
dried mixed herbs
1 tsp dried thyme
2 boneless and skinless chicken
breasts, cut into bite-sized chunks
1 leek, rinsed and finely chopped
black pepper

This is a great one-pan dish for a cold evening.

Pour 500ml of the stock into a flameproof casserole. Add the carrot, parsnip, mustard and thyme or mixed herbs and bring to a boil over a high heat. Boil for 8–10 minutes until the vegetables are starting to soften. Reduce the heat to low.

Using a potato masher, crush the vegetables so the parsnips mash slightly into the stock.

Add the chicken and leeks, cover the pan and simmer over a low heat for 15 minutes (be careful not to boil it or the chicken will toughen). Season with black pepper.

Serve the chicken casserole in warmed bowls with some spring greens.

Chicken tikka masala

Serves 2

Ingredients

7–8 heaped tbsp 0% fat natural Greek-style yoghurt
2 cloves garlic, peeled and finely chopped
5-cm root ginger, peeled and finely chopped
1 tbsp lemon juice, or juice of ½ lemon
1 tsp ground turmeric (optional)
½ tsp salt
300g boneless and skinless chicken thighs or breasts, cut into large chunks
1 tbsp coconut oil
1 medium onion, sliced
1 fresh red chilli, roughly chopped (remove seeds for a milder heat)
400g tin chopped tomatoes
25g creamed coconut
1 tsp garam masala
150ml boiling water
2 medium tomatoes, sliced
a handful of fresh coriander leaves and stalks, roughly chopped

VARIATION

For a lower-fat option, try 50g of coconut milk in place of the creamed coconut.

Indian isn't my favourite takeaway, but I do like it now and again. This recipe is a great way of adding variety.

Combine 4 heaped tablespoons of yoghurt with garlic, ginger, lemon juice, turmeric and salt to make a marinade. Add the chicken and mix it so it's well coated in the marinade. Cover and refrigerate for at least 30 minutes (it can be left overnight).

Heat half the coconut oil in a non-stick frying pan over a medium heat. Add the onion and chilli and fry for 6–8 minutes until the onion is golden.

Add the tomatoes, creamed coconut, garam masala and boiling water, lower the heat slightly and simmer for 6–8 minutes. You can leave the sauce like this, or use a stick blender to blitz it smooth.

Heat the remaining coconut oil in a second non-stick frying pan over a high heat. Once hot, add the chicken and fry for 5 minutes, turning halfway through to brown well on both sides. Add the sauce to the pan, stir and reduce the heat to low. Cover the pan with a lid and cook for 5 more minutes, adding a splash of water if it gets too dry, until the chicken is completely cooked through.

Serve with brown rice and garnish with the slices of tomato, coriander leaves and the remaining yoghurt.

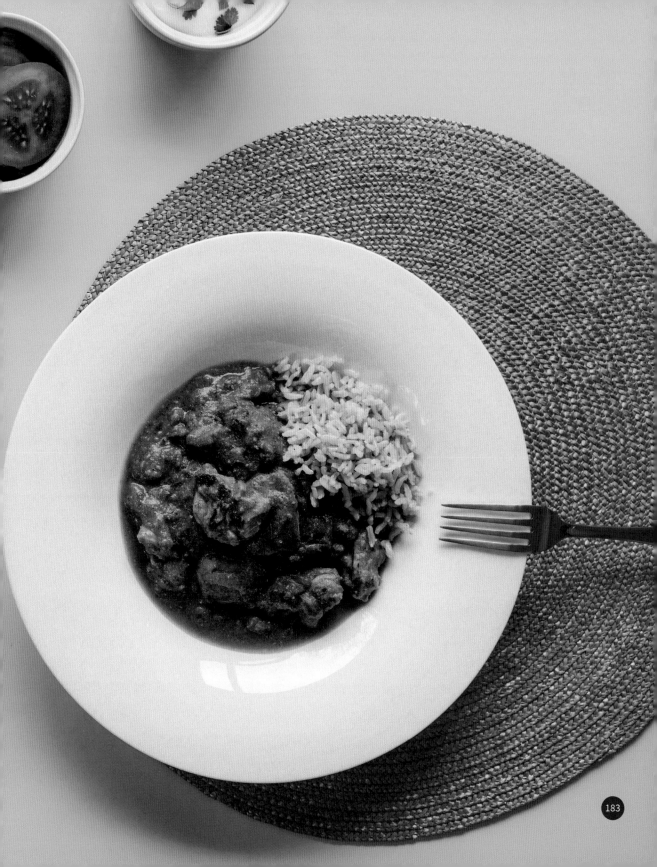

Sweet potato and tuna hash

Serves 2

This is a really easy dinner to have at the end of a busy day.

Ingredients

350g sweet potatoes, roughly chopped
2 tsp olive oil or coconut oil
6–8 spring onions, trimmed and thinly sliced
200g tin tuna in brine, drained (150g drained weight)
1 tbsp lemon juice or juice of ½ lemon (optional)
salt and black pepper

VARIATION

Add a finely chopped red, yellow or orange pepper or a handful of peas with the spring onions (defrost frozen peas quickly by putting them in a sieve and pouring over some boiling water). To give it more of a kick add a pinch of chilli flakes with the tuna.

Bring a large pan of salted water to the boil, add the sweet potato and boil over a medium heat for 15 minutes or until tender. Drain thoroughly then mash roughly (you don't want it too smooth) with some black pepper. Set aside.

Heat the olive oil or coconut oil in a non-stick frying pan over a medium-high heat. Add the spring onions and fry for 2 minutes.

Stir in the tuna and cook for a minute then add the sweet potato mash. Fry for 3–4 minutes, stirring once or twice, until heated through.

Stir in the lemon juice, if using, add some more black pepper and serve with Tenderstem broccoli or a baby spinach salad.

TIP: This is a great way to use up any leftover sweet potato mash or Root veg mash (see page 180) – you'll want about 250–300g.

Sweet potato and spinach tortilla

Serves 3

Because this can be kept in the fridge for up to two days it makes a great packed lunch the next day.

Ingredients
400g sweet potatoes, diced
6 medium free-range eggs
2 tsp coconut oil
1 medium yellow or red onion, chopped
100g spinach or baby spinach
salt and black pepper

VARIATION

This is good with a sliced red, yellow or orange pepper fried with the onion. Another alternative is to mix 1 teaspoon of pesto into the raw eggs. Or you could scatter 25g of crumbled feta on top before putting the tortilla under the grill.

Bring a large pan of salted water to the boil, add the sweet potato and boil over a medium-high heat for 10–12 minutes until just tender but not mushy. Drain thoroughly then return to the pan and put back on the heat for a minute to steam off any excess water. Set aside.

Preheat the grill to medium-high. Crack the eggs into a bowl, add salt and pepper and beat lightly with a fork.

Heat 1 teaspoon of the coconut oil in a non-stick frying pan over a medium heat. Add the onion and fry for 2–3 minutes until softened slightly then stir in the spinach and cook for a minute until wilted. Scrape these into the pan with the sweet potato.

Heat the remaining coconut oil in the frying pan and pour in the eggs. Spoon the sweet potato and onion mixture on top and gently swirl into the eggs. Reduce the heat to medium-low and cook for 5–7 minutes until set on the bottom and round the edges.

Put under the grill for 2–3 minutes or until puffed up and golden and the eggs are set. Serve hot or cold.

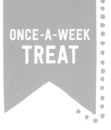

Asian prawn and noodle curry

Serves 2

Ingredients
100g dried rice noodles
1 tsp coconut oil
100ml coconut milk (from a tin or pouch)
50g red or green Thai curry paste
200g raw king prawns, defrosted if frozen
½ red pepper, seeds removed, thinly sliced
½ yellow pepper, seeds removed, thinly sliced
100ml boiling water
salt and black pepper

Because of the coconut milk this is a bit of a treat, so don't be tempted to have it too often!

Prepare the noodles according to the packet instructions. Set aside.

Heat the coconut oil and 3 tablespoons of coconut milk in a non-stick frying pan over a medium heat. Once bubbling add the curry paste and fry for 2 minutes. Add the prawns and season with salt and pepper then fry for 2–3 minuts until turning pink.

Stir in the peppers with the remaining coconut milk and the boiling water. Once bubbling, reduce the heat to low and simmer for a further 3 minutes.

Serve the noodles in bowls and spoon over the curry.

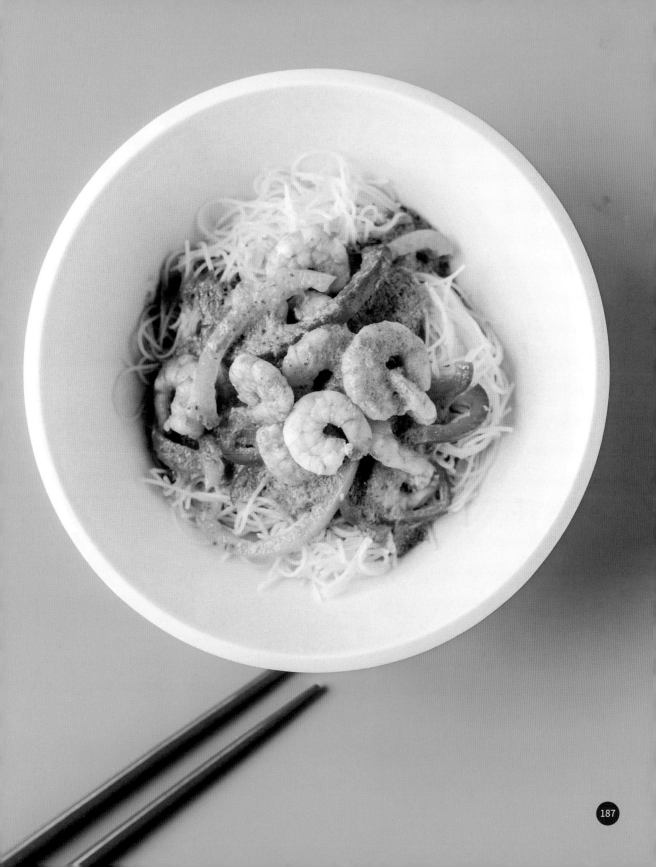

Chicken with tomatoes and mozzarella

Serves 2

Another simple but tasty dish using one of my favourite ingredients – mozzarella.

Ingredients
2 tsp olive oil
2 boneless and skinless chicken breasts
2 cloves garlic, peeled and thinly sliced
400g tin chopped tomatoes
½ tsp dried mixed herbs
60g mozzarella, sliced
sprig of flat leaf parsley, finely chopped (optional)
salt and black pepper

Preheat the grill to medium-high. Heat the olive oil in a non-stick frying pan over a medium heat. Add the chicken breasts, season with salt and pepper, and fry for 3 minutes on each side to brown slightly. Stir in the garlic and fry for a minute.

Stir in the tomatoes and herbs. Quarter-fill the empty tomato tin with water and add to the pan. Cook, bubbling gently, for 10 minutes then turn the chicken breasts, stir the sauce gently and cook for a further 5 minutes, or until the chicken is cooked through.

Lay the mozzarella slices on top of the chicken and put under a grill for 2 minutes until the cheese has melted. Sprinkle with fresh parsley, if using, and serve.

TIP: If you don't want to use the grill then just tear the mozzarella into the sauce and let it melt in for a minute or two.

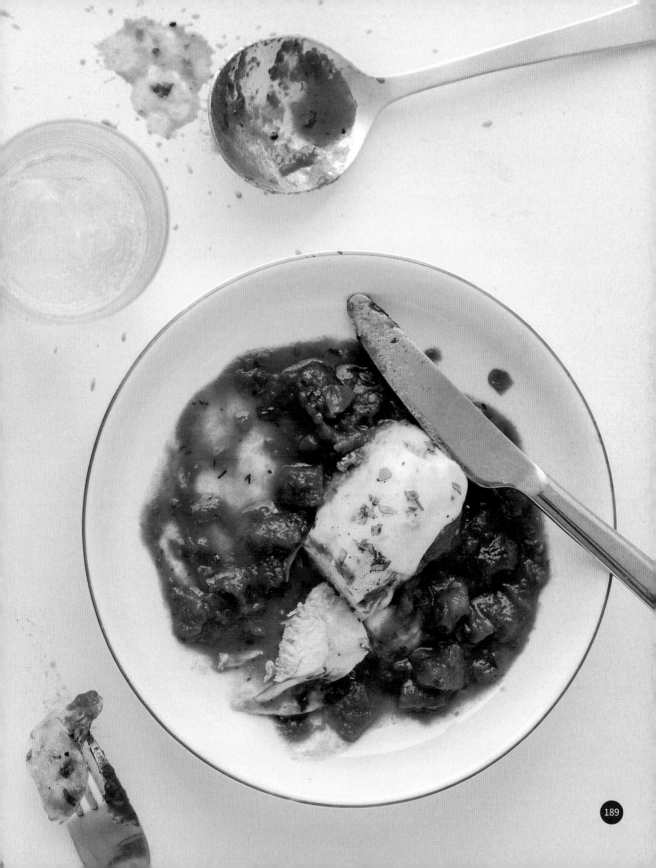

Sweet potato and salmon fishcakes

Serves 2

Because this recipe uses tinned salmon and frozen peas it's a store-cupboard staple you can always fall back on.

Ingredients

350g sweet potatoes, roughly chopped
170–200g tin pink salmon, drained
1 heaped tbsp tomato purée
1 tsp paprika or chilli powder
100g frozen peas, defrosted
lemon wedges
salt and black pepper

Preheat the oven to 200°C/gas 6 if planning to cook the fishcakes straight away.

Bring a large pan of salted water to the boil, add the sweet potato and boil over a medium heat for 15 minutes or until tender. Drain thoroughly then put back on the heat for a minute to steam off any excess water. Add all the remaining ingredients, except the lemon wedges, to the sweet potato and season with lots of pepper. Mix roughly with a fork, trying to keep some chunks in the potato and salmon (you ideally want the mixture a bit chunky rather than a smooth paste).

If you've got time, let the mixture cool then transfer to the fridge for an hour or so before making the fishcakes. Otherwise you can make them straight away. Divide the mixture into four and shape into rough fishcakes. Put on a non-stick baking tray.

Cook in the oven for 15–20 minutes until hot in the middle. Serve with lemon wedges to squeeze over the top and a mound of salad leaves.

TIP: This is a great way to use up any leftover sweet potato mash or Root veg mash (see page 180) – you'll want about 250–300g.

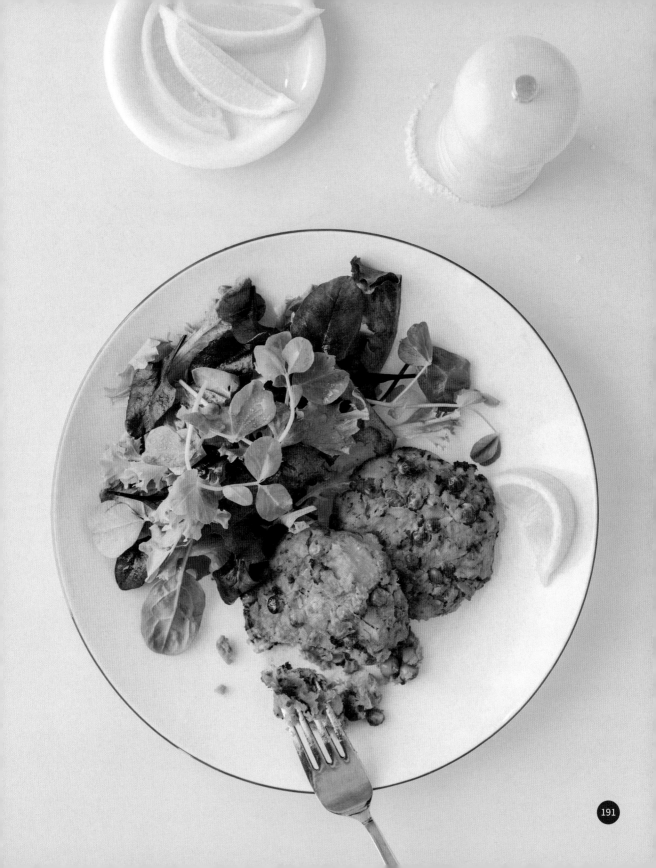

Thai-flavoured fishcakes

Serves 2

Ingredients

350g sweet potatoes, roughly chopped
170–200g tin pink salmon, drained
6 spring onions, trimmed and thinly sliced
1 fresh red or green chilli, finely chopped (remove seeds for a milder heat)
a handful of fresh coriander leaves and stalks, roughly chopped
lime wedges
salt and black pepper

And if you fancy your fishcakes a bit spicier…

Preheat the oven to 200°C/gas 6 if planning to cook the fishcakes straight away.

Bring a large pan of salted water to the boil, add the sweet potato and boil over a medium heat for 15 minutes or until tender. Drain thoroughly then put back on the heat for a minute to steam off any excess water.

To the pan of sweet potato, add the salmon, spring onions, fresh chilli and coriander. Mix roughly with a fork, trying to keep some chunks in the potato and salmon (you ideally want the mixture a bit chunky rather than a smooth paste). Season with salt and pepper.

If you've got time, let the mixture cool then transfer to the fridge for an hour or so before making the fishcakes. Otherwise you can make them straight away. Divide the mixture into four and shape into rough fishcakes. Put on a non-stick baking tray.

Cook in the oven for 15–20 minutes until hot in the middle. Serve with lime wedges to squeeze over the top and a mound of salad leaves.

Sweet potatoes stuffed with turkey, peppers, onion and goats' cheese

Serves 2

Ingredients
2 medium sweet potatoes (400g)
4 tbsp unsweetened almond milk,
oat milk or semi-skimmed milk
100g ready-cooked skinless turkey
breast or lean ham, all fat trimmed
off and finely chopped
1 red pepper, seeds removed, diced
1 medium red onion, diced
60g soft or crumbly goats' cheese,
feta or mozzarella, crumbled or diced
salt and black pepper

Everyone loves a jacket spud – this is the next best thing and a lot more healthy.

Prick the sweet potatoes a few times with a knife then microwave for 6–8 minutes until soft. If you don't have a microwave then cook in the oven at 200°C/gas 6 for 30–40 minutes.

Preheat the grill to medium-high.

Cut the cooked potatoes in half lengthways then scoop out the filling into a bowl. Put the skins into a baking dish. Mash the filling with the remaining ingredients, apart from the cheese.

Put the filling back into the potato skin and top with the cheese. Grill for 2–3 minutes until golden. Serve with a big green salad.

Roast lemon and mustard salmon

Serves 2

Ingredients

1 lemon, half cut into slices,
half for juice
2 salmon fillets, each weighing
125–150g, skin on
2 tsp wholegrain mustard
salt and black pepper

I really like the kick the mustard gives this recipe.

Preheat the oven to 200°C/gas 6.

Arrange the lemon slices in a non-stick roasting tin then sit the salmon fillets on top, skin side down. Squeeze the juice from the remaining lemon half over the fish. Season with salt and pepper then spread each fillet with 1 teaspoon of mustard. Pour 2 tablespoons of water into the roasting tin.

Cook the salmon in the oven for 12–15 minutes, or until just cooked through but not dry.

Serve with any juices spooned over and the Root veg mash (see page 180) if you're hungry, or you can simply have some green veg with it.

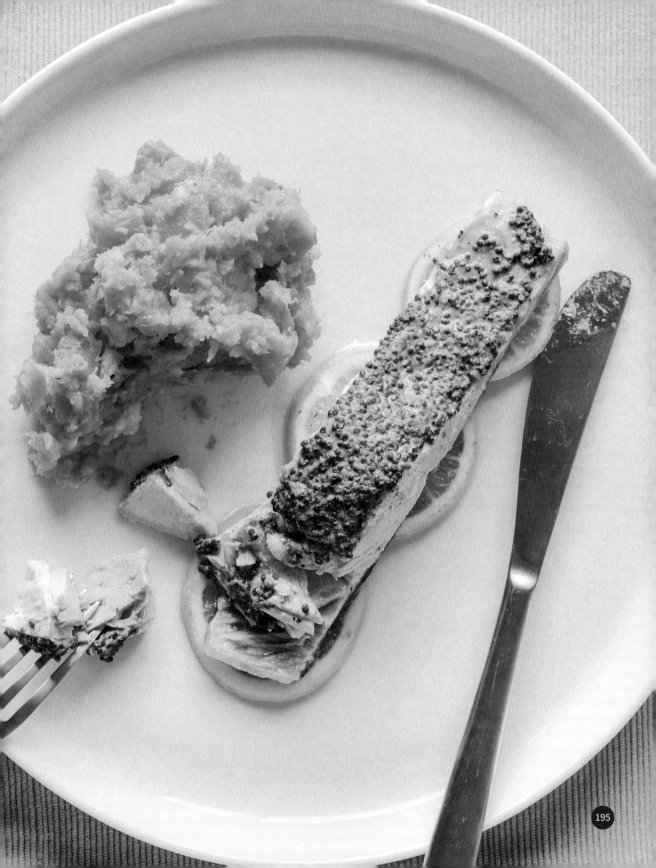

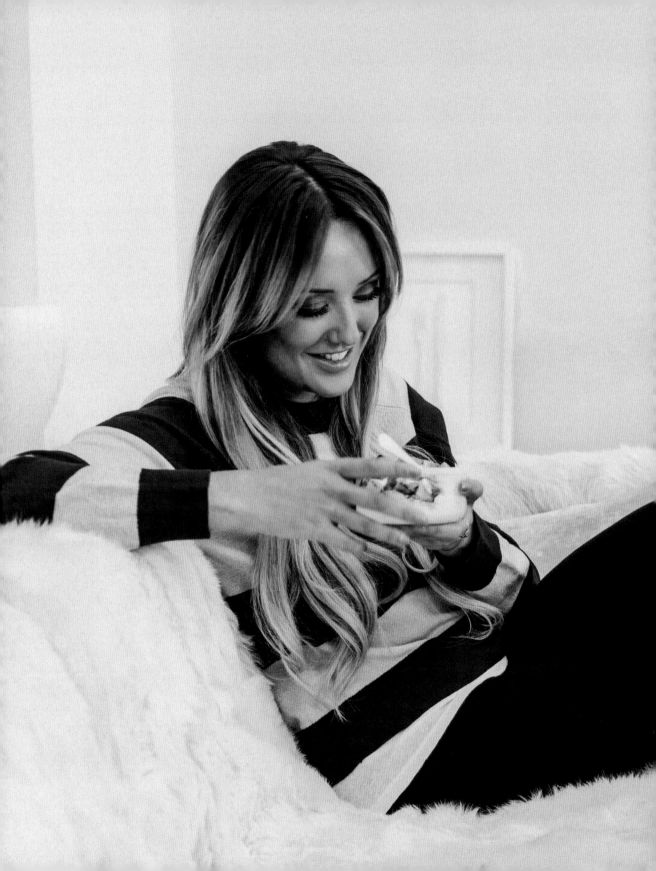

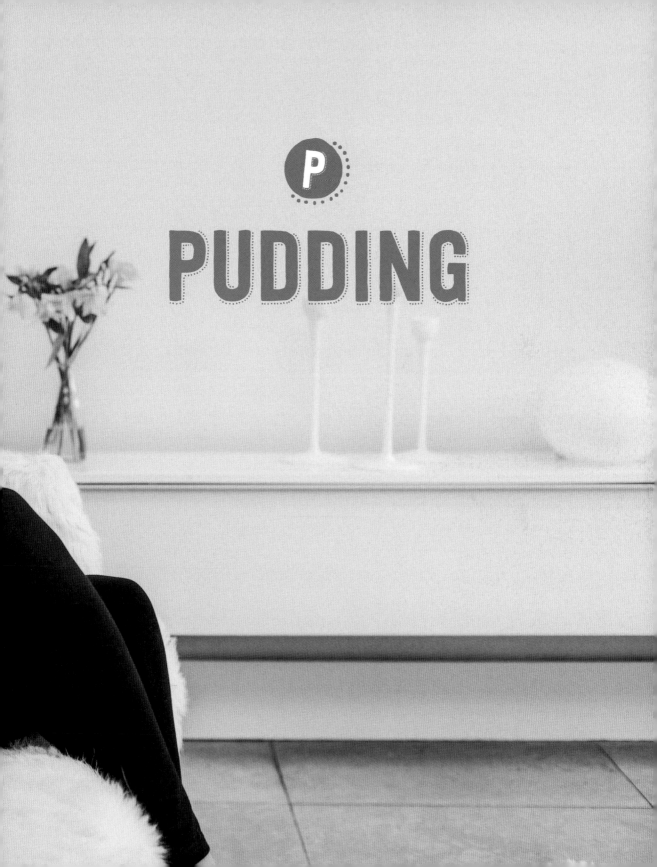

PUDDING

Healthier banoffee

Serves 1

If you feel like having something sweet, this is perfect – quick and healthier than a proper banoffee.

Ingredients
150g 0% fat natural
Greek-style yoghurt
1 tbsp crunchy or smooth peanut
butter (choose one with
no added sugar)
1 banana, peeled and sliced
2 oatcakes (20g), crumbled
1 small square dark chocolate (10g),
grated (optional)

Mix everything together in a bowl, saving some of the oatcake and the grated chocolate, if using, to sprinkle on top.

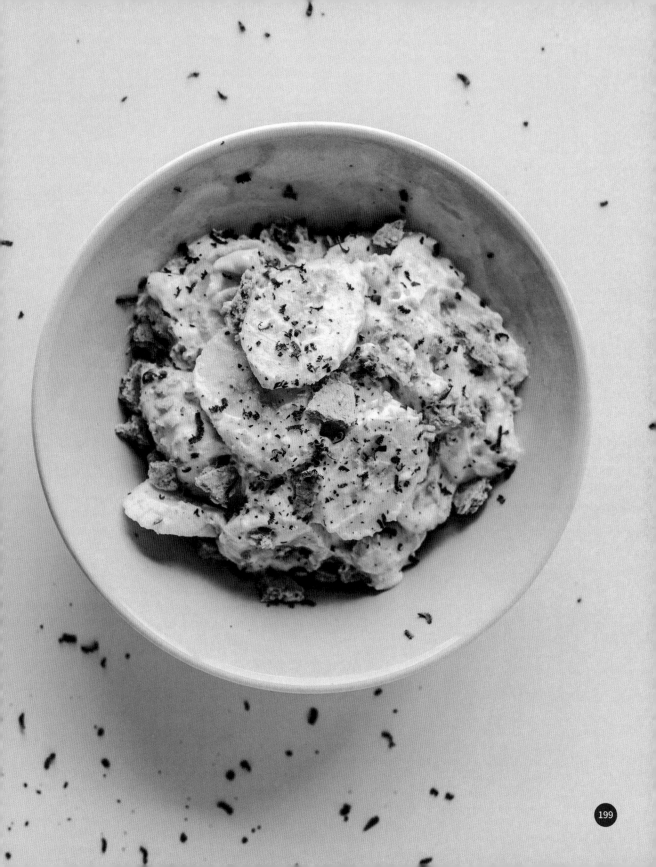

Sweet potato brownies

Makes 12

These are unreal – they actually taste like proper brownies.

Preheat the oven to 200°C/gas 6.

Put 1 tablespoon of coconut oil into a non-stick roasting tin and place in the oven for 2 minutes until melted. Tip the sweet potato and cinnamon into the hot tin and stir well to coat in the oil. Roast for 15–20 minutes until just tender. Scrape the sweet potato into a jug and use a stick blender to blitz it to a smooth purée. Set aside to cool slightly. Reduce the oven temperature to 170°C/gas 3.

In a small bowl or mug, mix 2 heaped tablespoons of cocoa power and the salt with the boiling water to form a paste. Set aside to cool.

Crack the eggs into a mixing bowl with the vanilla extract and honey. Use a handheld electric beater to whisk for a minute or two until pale in colour, or whisk vigorously by hand. Add the ground almonds, cocoa paste and sweet potato purée and beat well to combine. Lightly grease a baking tin (about 13 x 18cm, or 15cm square) with coconut oil. Tip the mixture into the tin and bake for 20 minutes. Remove and leave to cool in the tin before dusting with extra cocoa powder, if using, and cutting into twelve pieces.

TIP: These freeze, so no excuse for eating them all at once!

Ingredients

1 tbsp coconut oil, plus ½ tsp extra for greasing
300g sweet potatoes, diced
1 tsp ground cinnamon
2 heaped tbsp unsweetened cocoa powder, plus 1 tsp extra for dusting (optional)
a pinch of salt
60ml boiling water
2 medium free-range eggs
2 tsp vanilla extract
1 tbsp clear runny honey
120g ground almonds

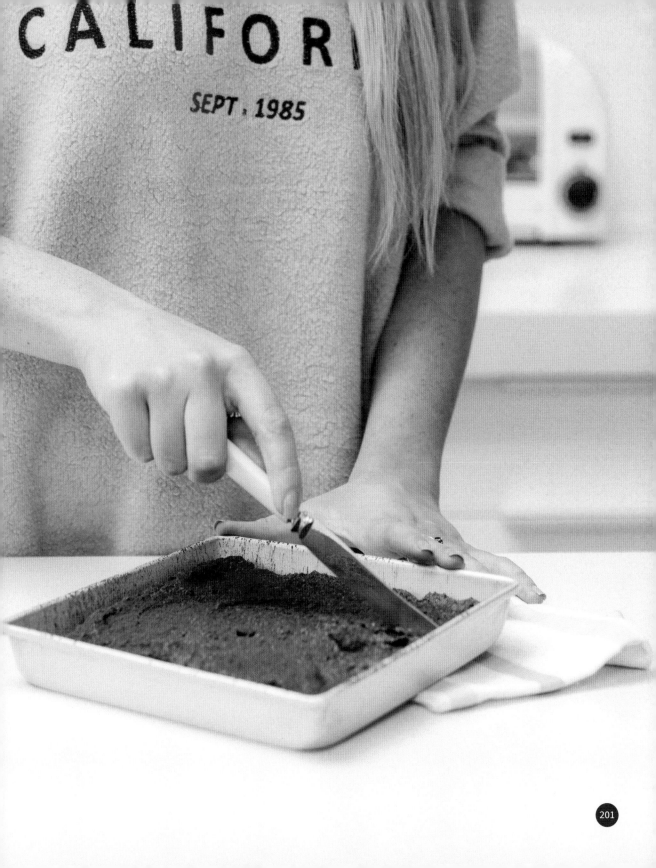

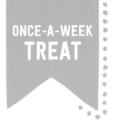
ONCE-A-WEEK
TREAT

Banana and dark chocolate ice cream

Serves 4

I don't think I need to sell this to you, girls. It's ice cream!

Tip everything, apart from the grated chocolate, into a food processor. Blitz to a smooth, creamy consistency. It will take a minute or two.

Serve straight away, topped with the grated chocolate, if using.

The texture is at its creamiest if eaten straight away, but otherwise transfer to a freezable container and freeze. Remove from the freezer 5–10 minutes before eating to soften slightly and give it a good mix before serving.

TIP: You need a sturdy food processor to make this ice cream. If it's struggling to blitz the bananas then add more milk.

Ingredients

3 large bananas, peeled, chopped and frozen (400g prepared weight)
100ml unsweetened almond milk, oat milk or semi-skimmed milk
½ tsp vanilla extract (optional)
2–3 tsp unsweetened cocoa powder
1 small square dark chocolate (10g), grated (optional)

VARIATION

You can add 2 tablespoons of smooth or crunchy peanut butter (choose one with no added sugar) or try melting two small squares of dark chocolate and swirling on top of the ice cream.

Oaty apple crumble

Serves 2

Ingredients
2 medium cooking apples, peeled,
cored and roughly chopped (300g
prepared weight)
½ tsp ground cinnamon
1 tsp clear runny honey
30g porridge oats
1 tbsp smooth peanut butter (choose
one with no added sugar)

A healthier and tastier take on your nana's favourite.

Preheat the oven to 200°C/gas 6.

Put the apple and 2 tablespoons of water in a saucepan.
Cover with a lid and cook over a medium heat for 10
minutes, stirring occasionally, until soft and fluffy. Stir in
the cinammon and honey.

Spoon the cooked apple into a roughly 20 x 10cm
ovenproof dish.

For the topping, mix the oats and peanut butter together
with your fingers. Scatter this over the apple and bake in
the oven for 15 minutes.

Serve while still hot.

Geordie mess

Serves 2

I'm not really a pudding person, but this – my own take on an Eton Mess – isn't too sweet. You could even have it for breakfast.

Ingredients

200g 0% fat natural Greek-style yoghurt
½ tsp vanilla extract (optional)
4 oatcakes (40g), crumbled
250g fresh berries (strawberries, raspberries)
½ tsp clear honey (optional)

Mix the yoghurt with the vanilla extract, if using.

Spoon half the yoghurt into a bowl and crumble over half the oatcakes and top with half the berries. Repeat with the remaining ingredients.

Serve in individual bowls and drizzle with the honey, if using.

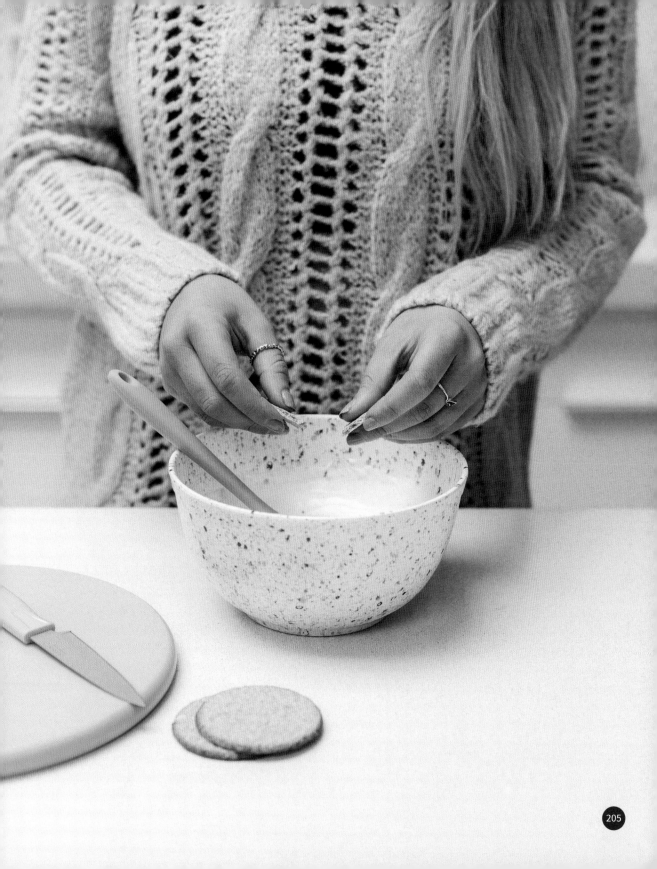

Frozen banana and chocolate pops

Makes 4

These are really fun and you can be dead creative with toppings. I think they are better than having an ice cream.

Ingredients
2 small bananas, peeled and cut in half through the equator
40g dark chocolate, broken into small pieces
1 tsp desiccated coconut
1 tsp chopped, toasted hazelnuts or flaked almonds, crumbled

Cover a baking tray with a piece of baking parchment or foil. Insert a lollipop stick or cocktail stick in the cut end of each banana half.

Melt the chocolate in the microwave, or in a heatproof bowl placed over a saucepan of barely simmering water. In both methods turn off the heat just before the chocolate is fully melted and leave it to melt in the residual heat – this stops it burning.

Dip the bananas in the melted chocolate to almost completely coat, then place them on the baking tray. Alternatively you can hold the bananas above a bowl and drizzle with the chocolate. Sprinkle immediately with either the coconut or the chopped nuts.

Freeze for at least half an hour before eating. Once frozen you can wrap each one in cling film and keep in the freezer for up to three weeks.

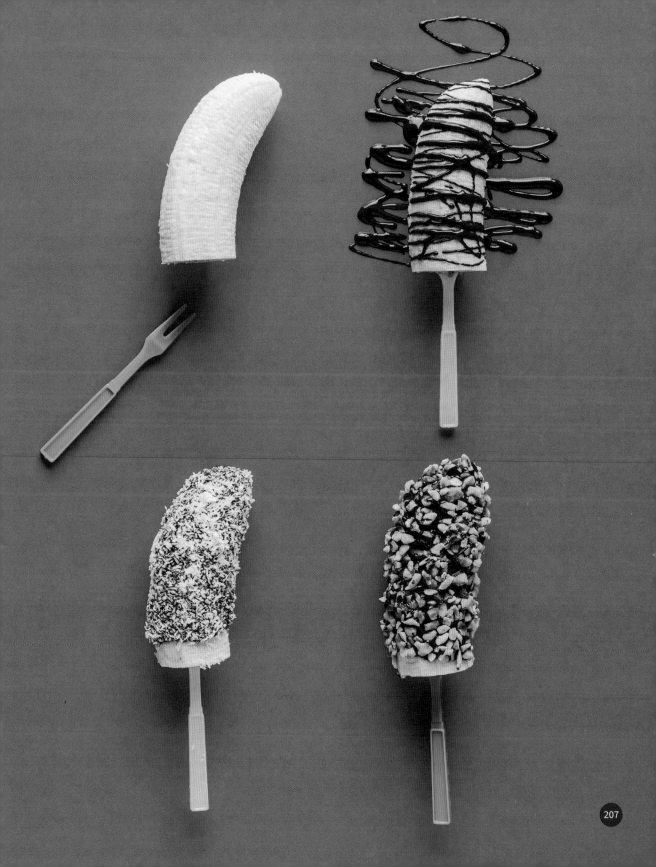

COCKTAILS

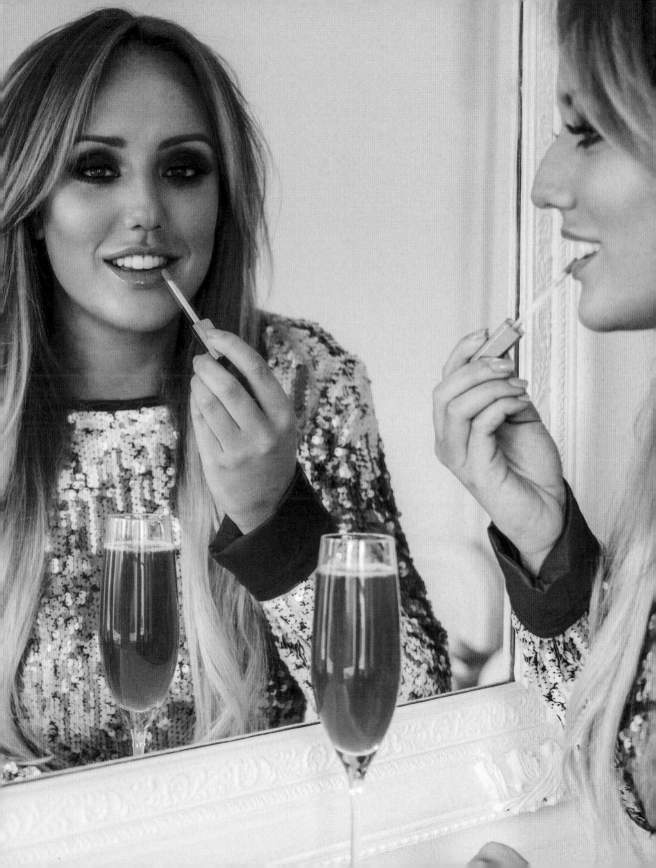

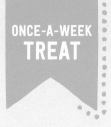

Frozen blueberry lime daiquiri

Serves 2

You can leave the booze out for a mocktail.

Ingredients
250g frozen blueberries
4–6 tbsp unsweetened 100%
pomegranate juice
4 tbsp vodka or white rum
1 lime, juice only
lime wedge (optional)

Put everthing except the lime wedge into a blender and blitz until very thick and smooth. Add more pomegranate juice if needed.

Pour into two glasses. Decorate with a lime wedge if you like. Serve with a straw.

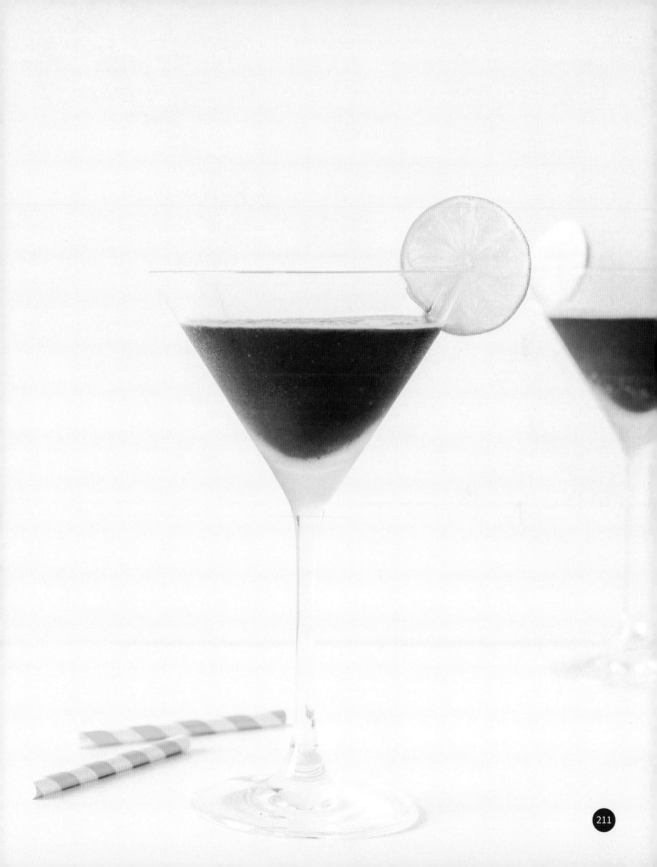

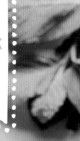

Vodka fruit cup

Serves 1

I make a big jug of this for my friends – just multiply the recipe by four or eight depending on how many us are there.

Ingredients
a handful of ice cubes
4 slices cucumber
2 strawberries, green stalks removed, chopped
2 slices lemon, chopped
2 slices orange, chopped
a sprig of fresh mint
2 tbsp vodka
75–100ml soda water

Put a few ice cubes in a tall glass. Add all of the fruit and the sprig of mint.

Pour over the vodka and top up with the soda. Stir gently and serve.

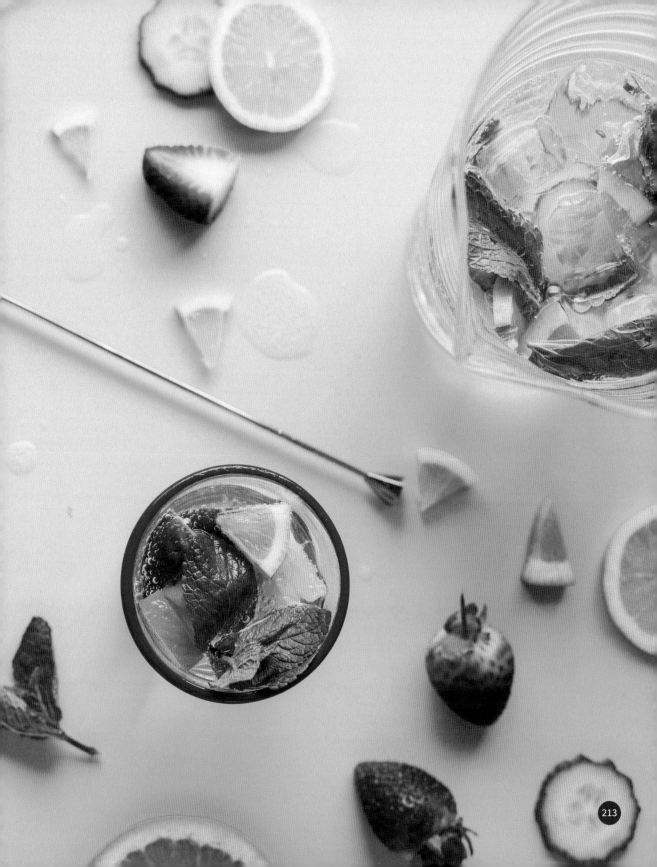

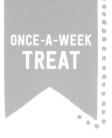

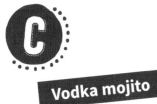

Vodka mojito

Serves 1

I like vodka whatever it's with, but this is better because it's with something that's never going to make you fat.

Ingredients

a handful of fresh mint leaves
½ lime, cut into wedges
a handful of ice cubes or crushed ice
2 tbsp vodka
75–100ml soda water

Put the mint and lime into a tall glass. Using the handle of a wooden spoon or a thin rolling pin, gently crush the lime and mint leaves together to bruise them slightly (this is called muddling).

Add the ice, pour over the vodka and top up with soda.

TIP: This is best made with crushed ice. Either put a handful of ice cubes in a sturdy plastic food bag and bash with a rolling pin, or blitz in a blender or sturdy food processor for a few seconds.

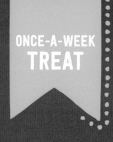

Vodka strawberries and peaches

Serves 2

At least with the peaches and strawberries you're getting some vitamins!

Ingredients
6–8 strawberries, green stalks removed, chopped into quarters
1 large peach, stone removed, roughly chopped
4 tbsp vodka
½ lime, juice only
a handful of ice cubes
75–100ml soda water

Put all of the ingredients, apart from the ice and soda, into a blender and blitz until smooth and thick.

Put some ice into two tall glasses. Pour in the peach mixture, top with a splash of soda and serve.

Pomegranate and grapefruit Prosecco

Serves 1

I love the flavour of pomegranate but I don't eat them because they've got loads of seeds in – which I don't like – so this is perfect for me.

Ingredients
1 tbsp grapefruit juice (from a carton or freshly squeezed)
3 tbsp unsweetened 100% pomegranate juice
100ml Prosecco

Pour the grapefruit and pomegranate juice into a champagne glass. Add the Prosecco and give a gentle stir to mix. Drink straight away!

TIP: You can buy 200ml bottles of Prosecco in most supermarkets now, which will make two glasses.

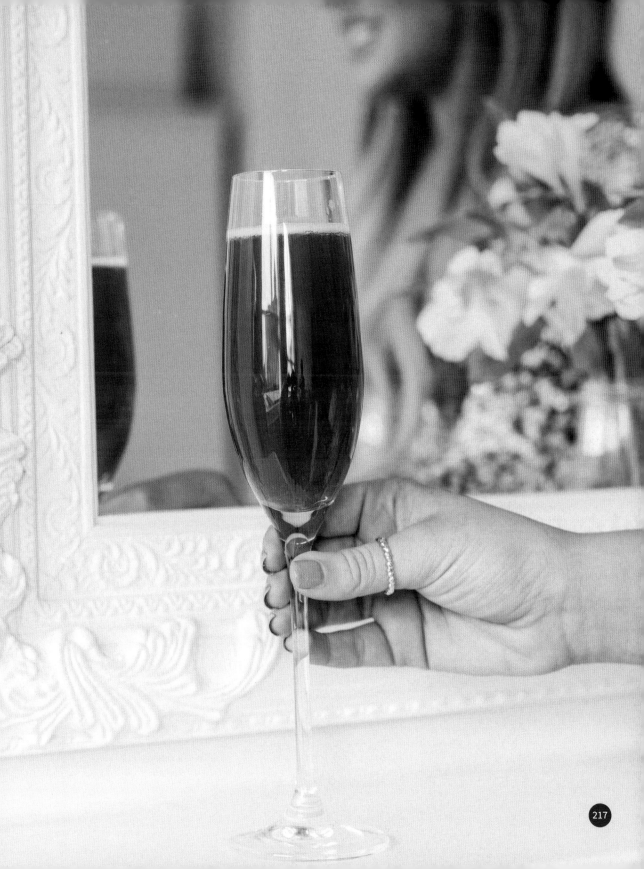

INDEX

THANKS TO...

Mam, Diddy and Nathaniel for supporting me endlessly, loving me unconditionally and also Mam for confronting me about my expanding belly and making the best soup in Sunderland.

Kate O'Shea, Martin O'Shea, Jade Reuben, Joe Foster, Jackie Christian, Felan Davidson and all the team at Bold Management. Sarah Emsley, Holly Harris, Emma Tait, Emma Rowley, Louisa Carter, Georgina Moore (Team Slick) and all at Headline for bringing my favourite recipes to life and giving me this opportunity to share them.

Jayne Irving, David Souter, Richard Callendar and Lara Gould: my fitness dream team, thank you for everything.

My amazing fans, thank you for following my journey, love you all!!

♡

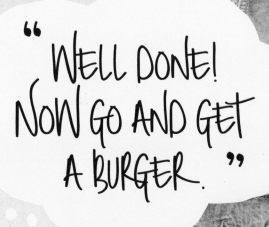